Take Control of Your Depression

Take Control of Your

DEPRESSION

Strategies to Help You
Feel Better Now

Susan J. Noonan, MD, MPH

Foreword by Jerrold F. Rosenbaum, MD,
and Timothy J. Petersen, PhD

Johns Hopkins University Press
Baltimore

Johns Hopkins University Press
2715 North Charles Street
Baltimore, Maryland 21218-4363
www.press.jhu.edu

Library of Congress Cataloging-in-Publication Data

Names: Noonan, Susan J., 1953– author.
Title: Take control of your depression : strategies to help you feel better now / Susan J. Noonan,
    MD, MPH ; foreword by Jerrold F. Rosenbaum, MD, and Timothy J. Petersen, PhD.
Description: Baltimore : Johns Hopkins University Press, 2018. | Series: A Johns Hopkins
    Press health book | Includes bibliographical references and index.
Identifiers: LCCN 2017056664 | ISBN 9781421426280 (hardcover : alk. paper) |
    ISBN 1421426285 (hardcover : alk. paper) | ISBN 9781421426297 (paperback : alk. paper) |
    ISBN 1421426293 (paperback : alk. paper) | ISBN 9781421426303 (electronic) |
    ISBN 1421426307 (electronic)
Subjects: LCSH: Depression, Mental—Popular works. | Depression, Mental—Treatment.
Classification: LCC RC537.N6625 2018 | DDC 616.85/27—dc23
LC record available at https://lccn.loc.gov/2017056664

A catalog record for this book is available from the British Library.

Special discounts are available for bulk purchases of this book. For more information, please contact Special Sales at 410-516-6936 or specialsales@press.jhu.edu.

Johns Hopkins University Press uses environmentally friendly book materials, including recycled text paper that is composed of at least 30 percent post-consumer waste, whenever possible.

Note to the reader: The information in this book should by no means be considered a substitute for the advice of qualified medical professionals. Mental diseases and disorders have a wide range of symptoms and clinical presentations. You should always consult qualified medical professionals for the diagnosis and treatment of mental diseases and disorders. All efforts have been made to ensure the accuracy of the information contained in this book as of the date of publication. The author and the publisher expressly disclaim responsibility for any adverse outcomes arising from the use or application of the information contained herein.

If you are thinking about suicide, you should immediately contact your health care provider, go to the nearest Emergency Department, or call 9-1-1.

Contents

Tables and Worksheets

Worksheets

Foreword

Despite many recent advances in options for assessment and treatment, depression remains a significant worldwide health problem. In the United States alone, up to 15 percent of individuals will suffer from depression at some point in their lifetime. Depression is now viewed as most often a recurrent illness, which requires lifelong management strategies.

The toll that depression exacts is massive, not only for the suffering individual but also for friends and family members. Many individuals diagnosed with depression are unable to work for periods of time, resulting in associated loss of productivity and disability. Rates of response to first-line treatments, while improved, remain unsatisfyingly low. Often a depressed individual requires a series of treatments before arriving at an acceptable therapeutic outcome. With the recent development of novel, cutting-edge interventions, the landscape of treatment options has become more complex. There are innovative therapeutics and novel targets on the horizon but, as yet a long-term aspiration, there is not "personalized" treatment selection soon to be available: thus, treatment will continue to require persistence and creativity on a patient-by-patient basis until relief is attained.

Susan J. Noonan, in this outstanding, updated edition of her 2013 book *Managing Your Depression*, tackles the challenge of providing to the general public a volume that provides a comprehensive "how to" guide for understanding and managing depression. Most impressive is the breadth of topics covered and pragmatic suggestions that will help engender hope that depression is a treatable illness. Among topics covered include behavioral strategies that are a core component of an overall depression treatment plan, cognitive strategies that are effective in "talking back" to negative thoughts, tips for accessing and maintaining an effective treatment team, effective ways to interact with loved ones during an episode of depression, and relapse prevention strategies.

Dr. Noonan's journey has been an inspiration to us at the Massachusetts General Hospital Department of Psychiatry. She has tirelessly proceeded through numerous psychosocial and medication treatments and has taught us much about perseverance, thinking outside the box, and the importance of not accepting anything short of becoming well. This volume, along with her other published works and speaking engagements, offers information and guidance that undoubtedly will help those suffering with depression.

Jerrold F. Rosenbaum, MD
Chief of Psychiatry, Massachusetts General Hospital
Stanley Cobb Professor of Psychiatry, Harvard Medical School

Timothy J. Petersen, PhD
Clinical Psychologist, Massachusetts General Hospital
Assistant Professor of Psychiatry, Harvard Medical School

Acknowledgments

This book is dedicated to a team of exceptional people who have made my life and this project possible. The superior clinical skills, extraordinary kindness, understanding, and perseverance of these professionals have been invaluable and have kept hope alive for me when I believed there was none. I owe my deepest thanks and gratitude to Drs. Andrew Nierenberg, Jonathan Alpert, Timothy Petersen, and Karen Carlson.

My family has been particularly generous and supportive in their own way, and for that I am most grateful. And my friends are the ones who have sustained me throughout. They deserve the highest praise for strength in friendship over a lifetime marked with a fluctuating illness. Enormous support has always come from my dear friend Ginger, who will be forever missed.

No book is published alone, and the amazing, insightful team of Jacqueline Wehmueller, Joe Rusko, and staff of Johns Hopkins University Press deserve particular recognition for guiding me through this remarkable journey.

Take Control of Your Depression

Introduction

The time you are feeling the worst is not the time to give up!
—ANDREW A. NIERENBERG

Some call it the blues or a storm in their head. William Styron called it darkness visible. Whatever the description, depression is a disorder of the mind and body that affects approximately 15 percent of the population at some point in their lives. Mood disorders such as major depression and bipolar disorder are conditions of the brain that involve a disturbance in one's mood or frame of mind. These conditions affect a person's thoughts, feelings, behaviors, relationships, activities, interests, and other aspects of life. Mood disorders can be quite overwhelming.

The symptoms of major depression and bipolar disorder are often remitting and relapsing. This means that the symptoms come and go over time; they may improve or go away and then return at some later time. The pattern is unique for each person and difficult to predict. You may experience symptoms for a long time, just as people who have diabetes or high blood pressure often do. The important thing to remember is that mood disorders are treatable, and that you can learn to manage yours and *thrive*.

One of the most common symptoms of major depression and bipolar disorder is difficulty with concentration and focus. In Styron's book, he eloquently described a state of confusion, failure of mental focus, lapse of memory, and muddied thought processes, familiar to many who have depression. Experiencing these symptoms may make it challenging for you to read, pay attention to a conversation or TV show, or remember simple things. Although advice on how to manage a mood disorder can be found in many textbooks, self-help books, and websites, a person who has depression may find some of these resources difficult to follow and absorb. Books and articles with long, involved text can be overwhelming to a person in the midst of depression. These difficulties are symptoms of the disease, not indications of your intelligence. Because of these symptoms, learning to manage depression requires a different approach.

So, I carefully targeted the problems of concentration and focus in writing this book. It was designed to focus on practical, day-to-day ways to manage your illness. The suggestions presented are things you can do on your own, in addition to receiving professional health care or mental health services. My goal is to provide you with core information that is brief and to the point. The basics of managing your depression or bipolar disorder are broken down into several sections, with skill sets and exercises you can do one at a time. My perspective in writing is that of a physician who has treated many patients and who also has personal experience living with the illness. Having been in the depths of a mood disorder, I understand what information is most helpful to manage the illness and how it is best received.

I gathered the information presented here over time from various educational resources, psychoeducational programs, seminars, expert health care providers, and personal patient experience. If you suffer from mood disorders, you can use this book in two main ways:

1. As an educational source to better understand and manage your illness: You need to have specific knowledge and skills to respond to an illness like depression so that you can avoid its worsening, be able to recover, and prevent recurrences. Managing your mood disorder in an informed way can help you function better and stay well. People who participate actively in their own care and who work to manage their mood disorder have a better chance of recovery and of staying well.
2. As a workbook, a set of skills and exercises to use along with input, advice, and treatment from your therapist and treatment team. This book is not intended to replace your treatment professionals.

I advise you to go slowly. Review one section at a time and keep in mind that you may need to review it more than once. People who have depression experience various clinical signs and symptoms in a pattern that is unique to each of them. Look for the material that applies to your own experiences over time. You may find some of the exercises to be starting points for discussions in your therapy sessions. Work with your therapist to determine the most helpful educational and exercise tools for you. It's worth repeating—people who participate actively in their care have a better chance of recovery and of staying well.

Who is this book written for? Everybody and anybody who has a mood disorder. Many of the recommendations, especially the basics of mental health (see chapter 1), are likely to be helpful even if you don't have a mental health condition. But these basics are particularly beneficial to those who do have an illness. The ideas are simple, practical ways to take control of your health. You don't need fancy resources to get adequate sleep, nutrition, and daily physical exercise like walking around the block, or to add a structure and routine to your day. These steps are considered part of your self-management of the illness, useful strategies in addition to whatever professional mental health therapy is available to you. And they're backed by science. We don't all live in areas close to mental health treatment centers. Some of us who do may not know how to gain access to the resources we need or are reluctant to go for professional treatment. The steps in my book will help you lay the foundation to build a healthy emotional state.

Some of you who read this book may find that a few of the ideas feel familiar to you. You might think, "Yeah, so what, already heard that!" For others, these may be brand new concepts. In either case, I present the ideas to you because *knowing* that something is good for you is not the same as *doing* it. There's a difference between intellectually knowing something and being able to take the steps when depressed to do that same thing. Taking action is the hard part and our greatest challenge. One way to help yourself get motivated and actually do something is to understand the reasons behind it. That's where this book becomes helpful to you. I offer suggestions backed by the medical evidence as reported in sound scientific studies, filtered by knowing what has been helpful to me and others based on real personal experience.

I begin in chapter 1 with the mental health basics, the essential things we all need to do daily to maintain emotional health and stability. The basic steps include maintaining a regular pattern of sleep, diet, exercise, medications, and social contacts; keeping a routine and structure to your day; and avoiding isolation. These fundamental actions can be especially challenging when you are managing a mood disorder because the symptoms of depression often interfere with your ability to do them.

In the second chapter, I give an overview of the mood disorders called major depression and bipolar disorder. This chapter also includes a brief discussion of depression in women, men, adolescents, the elderly, and those who have chronic illness or cancer; as well as information about depression and anxiety, the stigma of mood disorders, and fatigue and depression. There is a comprehensive table of the real-life symptoms of major depression and bipolar disorder, as well as a daily Mood Chart to track your symptoms.

Next, chapter 3 discusses the common obstacles in depression that often trip us up. These include being consumed by depression, having a fear of recovery, and rumination. Having an awareness and understanding of these potential barriers to recovery is an important step in achieving wellness.

Chapter 4 presents the concept of *defining your baseline*. Your baseline is your healthy inner self, something that appears to be lost during severe depression, even if only temporarily. In managing depression, you have to find a way to stay connected to your baseline healthy person, your inner sense of yourself. This baseline can be extraordinarily helpful to draw on during your recovery. This chapter also includes exercises to help you identify and define your baseline self.

Chapter 5 begins with an overview of treatment for mood disorders, including talk therapy, medications, and inpatient care. It addresses the questions, *What do I do if I'm reluctant to seek treatment?* and *What if I can't afford treatment?* Chapter 5 continues with a discussion of your relationship with your therapist, followed by what you need to know to manage your depression or bipolar disorder. It is important to use both professional treatment and self-management techniques to achieve the best recovery from your illness. Managing depression means learning about the illness and its symptoms as well as developing effective strategies to respond to your symptoms. It requires that you monitor your symptoms, challenge negative thoughts, use problem-solving techniques, make adjustments, and avoid negative behaviors.

The concept of wellness and well-being is addressed in chapter 6, "What Is the Goal?" Here, I present the idea that it is not enough to be free of mood disorder symptoms. The goal is to be well. Wellness is not the absence of symptoms but the presence of several life skills, as described by psychologist C. D. Ryff, which I review for you in this chapter. It *is* possible for someone who has depression to experience wellness.

In chapter 7, you will find an overview of relapse prevention. Relapse prevention is an effective daily approach to help you minimize the chance of a relapse (return of symptoms) and to help you stay well. This chapter also provides ways to identify your depression warning signs and triggers as well as an Action Plan for Relapse Prevention to use when an important change in your emotional health happens. It concludes with tips on what to do if you feel suicidal.

Chapter 8 is a presentation of cognitive behavioral therapy (CBT), a specific type of talk therapy that addresses the connection between your thoughts, feelings, and behaviors. CBT is particularly useful in depression when your thoughts are distorted, negative, and causing you distress. This form of therapy helps to identify and change distorted thinking patterns, inaccurate beliefs, and unhelpful behaviors that are common in depression.

Included in this chapter are sample CBT exercises for you to use to challenge and change dysfunctional thinking patterns.

I explore in chapter 9 some life strategies to get you through the tough times. These skills often fade during depression, so you may need to review and polish up on them. This chapter covers coping and stress, mindfulness, distress tolerance, communication skills, talking with your doctor, and tips you can share with your families and friends.

In chapter 10, I discuss strategies for dealing with family and friends, which can often be stressful and affect your illness. The advice applies to a wide range of people from those in your closest circle to casual acquaintances or your supervisor at work. Here, you will find ideas on when and how to disclose your illness, as well as tips on managing important relationships. Following that is a section on how to survive the holidays with difficult family members.

Chapter 11 describes how it looks and feels to manage your depression by incorporating the recommendations throughout this book into your daily life. Chapter 12 is a collection of thoughtful advice and resources for your review, including a section on technology and mental illness, reliable and recommended internet sites, and books of interest. Then check out the list of books and websites written by others who have learned to cope with and manage their illness. Next is a concluding chapter, which is rounded out by an appendix of medications used in mood and sleep disorders, a glossary of important terms used in the book, references, and an index.

Mental Health Basics

Action precedes motivation.
—ROBERT J. MCKAIN

THE BASIC STEPS

The basics of mental health are the essential actions we all need to engage in every day to maintain emotional health and stability. They are especially important when you are trying to manage a mood disorder. The basic steps include

maintaining a regular pattern of sleep, a healthy diet, and regular
physical exercise;
taking prescribed medications;
keeping up with social contacts and avoiding isolation; and
having a routine and structure to your day.

The steps, summarized in box 1.1, are your foundation for a healthy emotional life. On this foundation, you will build the components of your treatment plan. These may feel like common-sense recommendations that you've heard before, but they are essential to controlling your symptoms. Controlling your symptoms in this way improves the quality of your life. When you follow these steps regularly, you decrease your vulnerability to fluctuations, or changes, in your mood disorder symptoms. Taking care of your overall self is important to your general health and to preserving your emotional balance and strength. It also boosts your resilience. This helps you to recover more quickly from setbacks or episodes of depression if they do occur.

Following these fundamental steps can be especially challenging when you are struggling to manage a mood disorder because the symptoms of depression often interfere with your ability to actually *do* the steps. As an example, the symptoms of fatigue, poor appetite, and lack of interest can make it difficult to do the grocery shopping and cooking necessary to follow

---

BOX 1.1. The Basics of Mental Health

Treat any physical illness.

Sleep:

- Aim for 7 to 8 hours of sleep each night.
- Keep a regular sleep routine.
- Follow sleep hygiene principles to promote restorative, restful sleep.
- Use a sleep diary to track sleep patterns.

Maintain a healthy diet and nutrition:

- Eat balanced, healthy meals regularly, 3 times a day.
- Do not use alcohol, street drugs, or excessive caffeine.

Medication:

- Take all medications as prescribed, even if you are feeling better.
- Discuss with your physician all over-the-counter medications, herbs, and other supplements you take.

Exercise regularly (as able); balance cardiovascular, stretching, and strengthening activities.

Maintain regular social contacts and connections with others.

Avoid isolation.

Follow a daily routine and structure your time.

---

a healthy diet. To meet this particular challenge, you might find the strategies given in table 1.1 helpful.

You'll learn more about these tips in this and the following chapters. Don't wait until you feel like doing something to start. Just do it as best as you can now and the motivation for doing it will follow. Many people with depression have found that to be so. Keep trying despite the difficulty and give yourself credit for the effort.

SLEEP AND DEPRESSION

Sleep problems, including insomnia, often occur during an episode of major depression or bipolar disorder. When depressed, you may sleep a lot but still feel tired. You may sleep too little or have interrupted sleep, with frequent

TABLE 1.1. **Strategies to Help You Follow a Healthy Diet**	
STRATEGY	**EXAMPLES**
Plan for what you have to do.	• Shop at a time of day when you have more energy. • Ask a friend to help you with the groceries.
Break down tasks of daily life into small steps.	• Follow simple recipes, five ingredients or fewer. • Write down your grocery list, meal by meal. • Only buy the items you need or use frequently.
Pace yourself.	• Cook healthy foods in large batches on days you have more energy. • Freeze some for later meals when you may be too fatigued to cook.

awakenings during the night. You may have trouble falling asleep, or you may wake up too early. The quality of your sleep may be affected so that you don't feel rested or restored the next day. Without enough sleep you may become irritable and have difficulty concentrating and doing small tasks. In contrast, in bipolar disorder with mania or hypomania, you may feel that you don't need very much sleep at all, that you are energized and awake during normal sleep times.

Why does sleep matter to your *mental health*? Sound sleep optimizes brain function and has a positive effect on your mood disorder. A change in the amount or quality of sleep will affect your illness. For example, periods of insufficient or poor-quality sleep can worsen your depression or bring on your bipolar illness. A consistent period of getting a good night's sleep can help improve your mood.

Why does sleep matter to your *physical health*? Prolonged insomnia, especially when sleeping fewer than 6 hours per night, is thought to be associated with an increased risk of heart disease, high blood pressure, and diabetes. If you can improve your sleep quality and quantity, these general physical conditions are potentially preventable. This is why it's important to get control of your sleep.

Changes in your sleep may or may not be fully under your control. They may be related to a physical condition such as sleep apnea or extreme stress. Sleep difficulties may be warning signs or symptoms of your worsening mood disorder, which you and your treatment team can recognize and address. Sleep disruption may also be related to environmental conditions, such as noise level, excess light, or extremes in room temperature. The good news is that you can control some things to help yourself achieve a good night's sleep. Recommended treatment for long-standing insomnia includes two main approaches: cognitive behavioral therapy and sedating medication.

Cognitive behavioral therapy for insomnia (CBT-I), a type of talk therapy, is considered the first-line treatment for sleep problems. It addresses the dysfunctional thoughts, beliefs, and behaviors about sleep that contribute to a persistent sleep problem. CBT-I includes sleep restriction, cognitive therapy to restore and maintain reasonable expectations about sleep, relaxation therapy, and sleep hygiene. Sleep hygiene helps to reduce behaviors that interfere with sleep or increase your excitability or stimulation around bedtime.

The appendix provides a brief listing of common drugs that might be used for sleep and other mental health problems.

SLEEP HYGIENE

Sleep hygiene refers to the personal habits and environmental (home) conditions that affect your sleep. Good sleep habits can help improve your sleep, which in turn will help improve your mood. So it is important to maintain good sleep habits and a consistent sleeping and waking pattern in a bedroom environment that favors sound sleep. Sleep hygiene recommendations, adapted from the American Academy of Sleep Medicine, are listed in box 1.2. One of the essential steps in managing your mood disorder is to follow these recommendations as best as you can. Speak with your doctor if you are still having sleep problems after practicing good sleep hygiene.

You might now be wondering, *What is enough sleep for me?* The amount of sleep required by a person depends in part on age. It varies from infancy, through childhood, to older age. The average amount of sleep required by healthy adults is 7 to 8 hours per night. "Enough sleep" is the amount that makes you feel physically and mentally rested, sharp, not irritable, and able to concentrate, focus, and correctly do small motor tasks.

BOX 1.2. Sleep Hygiene

Recommendations to improve your sleep:

- Keep the same bedtime and wake-up time every day, including weekends. Set an alarm clock if necessary. Get up and out of bed at the same time even if you've had a bad night's sleep.

- Avoid napping during the day.

- Develop a relaxing sleep ritual before bedtime. Create downtime in the last 2 hours before going to bed and avoid overstimulation, such as family arguments, excess noise, vigorous activity, or violent TV shows or video games.

- Limit exposure to bright light in the evenings.

- Turn off all electronic devices at least 30 minutes before bedtime, including smartphones, tablets, and computers.

- Try going to bed only when you are sleepy.

- Avoid watching the clock. Turn the clock away from you.

- Avoid lying in bed unable to fall asleep and feeling frustrated. If you are not asleep after 20 to 30 minutes, get out of bed. Relax and distract your mind with a quiet activity in another room (music, reading), then return to bed when you are sleepy.

- Relaxation exercises before bedtime may be helpful. Examples include progressive muscle relaxation, deep breathing, guided imagery, yoga, and meditation.

- Designate a specific "worry time" earlier in the day or evening to sort out problems you may have. Writing down reminders for the next day is a good way to clear your mind before bed.

- Use your bed and bedroom only for sleep, sex, or occasional illness. Eliminate nonsleep activities in bed, using another room for reading, watching TV, working, and eating.

- Limit how much caffeine you have during the day, and avoid its use after 12:00 noon. Note that coffee, tea, colas, cocoa, chocolate, and some medications contain caffeine.

- Avoid or limit the use of nicotine (tobacco) and alcohol during the day and avoid their use within 4 to 6 hours of bedtime.

- Avoid large meals before bedtime, but don't go to bed hungry. If needed, have a light snack.

- Exercise regularly. Avoid strenuous exercise within 4 to 6 hours of bedtime.

(*continued*)

- Create a bedroom environment that favors sound sleep. A comfortable bed in a dark, quiet room is recommended. Minimize light, noise, and extremes in room temperature (hot or cold) in the bedroom. Room-darkening shades, curtains, earplugs, or a sound machine may be helpful.
- Speak with your physician if you are having continued difficulty with sleep, including falling asleep, staying asleep, and early or frequent awakenings.

Source: Adapted in part from the American Academy of Sleep Medicine, "Healthy Sleep Habits," updated February 9, 2017, www.sleepeducation.org/essentials-in -sleep/healthy-sleep-habits.

How do you know *how much sleep* you are really getting and what your *sleep patterns* are? Most people tend to underestimate the amount of sleep they had. One way to know is to keep track of your sleep for several weeks with a sleep diary (table 1.2). A sleep diary is a chart where you record

- your bedtime
- how long it took to get to sleep
- the number of times you woke up during the night
- how long you stayed awake (duration of awakening)
- the time you are finally awake and out of bed in the morning

Fill it out first thing in the morning for several weeks and then share it with your doctor(s). Keeping a sleep diary helps you and your treatment team understand your sleep patterns. It is used to track your progress and response to therapy, and it provides valuable information used in making treatment decisions. It also helps you to stick with good sleep hygiene habits.

DIET AND NUTRITION

You have probably heard that it's important to eat a nutritious and varied diet to keep your body and vital organs working properly. Did you know that this is also true for your brain? Food is the fuel that keeps your body and your brain functioning optimally. This includes managing your emotions and mood disorder. If you eat healthy food on a regular schedule you provide continuous fuel to your body and brain. Feed your body, feed your brain.

When you stray from a healthy regular diet you become vulnerable to mood changes. You may become irritable and fatigued, and your brain may not function very well. If you skip meals or eat in response to emotional cues, you tend to overeat when you do not need to, and this affects your mood state.

Here's how it works. When you eat starchy or sweet foods (called *carbohydrates*) or alcohol, the body digests it, breaking it down into a sugar called *glucose*. Carbohydrate foods include bread, pasta, rice, beans, peas, corn, sweet potatoes, potatoes, winter squash, and of course cookies, cake, pastries, and other baked goods. Glucose travels around in your bloodstream so that your cells can use it for energy. Insulin, a hormone made by the body, carefully controls the amount of glucose in your blood.

After you eat, the amount of glucose becomes high, and the body releases insulin in response to bring the glucose back down to "normal" levels. If you binge or eat too many carbohydrates, the body makes too much insulin and your blood sugar swings from high to low. This creates havoc with your mood and energy level. You become fatigued, irritable, and anxious, and you have poor concentration and mood swings. The goal is to keep your glucose levels steady throughout the day by eating a diet balanced with moderate and equal amounts of carbohydrate and lean protein at each meal. Well-balanced meals contain 3 to 5 ounces of protein (depending on your physical size); healthy snacks contain 1 to 2 ounces. Protein, fat, and fiber (in order of effectiveness) keep you full and prevent quick rises and falls in blood sugar. This keeps your blood sugar (glucose) in the optimal range for hours after you eat, and helps you feel good, energized, and clear headed, with a better mood.

> Eating well-balanced healthy meals is one way of taking care of yourself that you have control over. It can make a positive difference in your mental health.

A visual image of this concept is displayed in figure 1.1, which was created by Marc O'Meara, RD, LD, CDE, a senior nutritionist at the Brigham and Women's Hospital Department of Nutrition, Boston, Massachusetts. The graph shows, on the dotted line, the effect on your blood sugar of eating a high-carb meal or snack, with many ups and downs. In contrast, the solid line shows how a well-balanced meal or snack keeps your blood sugar in a steady range. Sometimes a picture like this is worth a thousand words!

The body makes other hormones that have an active role in the digestive process. *Leptin* is a hormone secreted by fat cells that signals to the brain that you ate enough (giving you a sense of fullness). Chronic stress and overeating can lead to leptin resistance, which means you never know when you're full. A third hormone, *ghrelin*, stimulates the appetite and lowers leptin, so

Day	Bedtime	SOL* (time it takes to fall asleep)	Number of times you woke up during the night	How long, total, were you awake during the night?	Latest time awake	What time did you get out of bed?	Total time asleep
MONDAY							
TUESDAY							
WEDNESDAY							
THURSDAY							
FRIDAY							
SATURDAY							
SUNDAY							

TABLE 1.2. **Sleep Diary**

Source: Adapted from National Institutes of Health and National Heart, Lung, and Blood Institute, *Your Guide to Healthy Sleep* (Bethesda, MD: NHLBI, 2011), www.nhlbi.nih.gov/files/docs/public/sleep/healthy_sleep.pdf.

*SOL = sleep onset latency.

Did you nap during the day? For how long?	Medications	Exercise	Notes / medication changes

FIGURE 1.1. **The effect of meal composition on blood sugar, hunger, and weight**

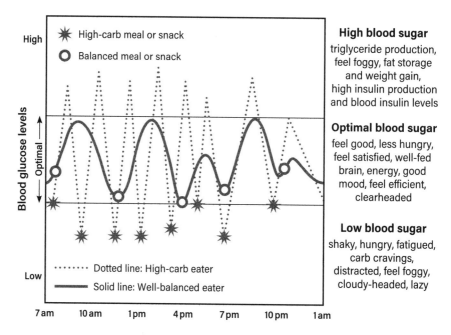

Based on original graph developed by Marc C. O'Meara, RD, LD, CDE, Brigham and Women's Hospital, Boston, Massachusetts.

you end up eating more. Poor-quality sleep increases ghrelin and triggers the brain to increase the appetite. Now you can see how changes in the stress and sleep patterns in your life have an effect on how your body uses the food you eat.

Several research studies have shown an association between particular eating patterns and mental health. Some diets are thought to be associated with different rates of depression. For example, a Western diet is associated with increased rates of depression, while a Mediterranean diet is linked with decreased rates (table 1.3). It is not known whether a poor-quality diet is a result of the appetite changes and inertia that accompany depression or whether it causes those symptoms—perhaps both are true. Other studies have shown the significance of the supplements folate, vitamin B12, and omega-3 fatty acids in the diet, but this is a complex discussion beyond the scope of this book. Talk with your doctor about whether you need to take any dietary supplements for your depression.

A healthy eating pattern is valuable for additional reasons. Improving your brain's nutritional status may increase the effectiveness of antidepressant medications. A healthy diet can also counteract the frustrating side

DIET	EXAMPLES	MOOD
TABLE 1.3. **Western Diet versus Mediterranean Diet**		
Western diet: high in saturated fats and processed, fried, and sugary foods	Burgers, shakes, fries, chips, junk food	Associated with a high rate of depression
Mediterranean diet: fresh, balanced, and less-processed foods	Fruits, vegetables, legumes, fish, lean protein, whole grains, olive oil, nuts	Associated with a lower rate of depression

effects of having a mood disorder. For example, depression, lack of activity, sleep problems, and many medications prescribed for mood disorders have the potential to increase body weight. This means that you have to be particularly vigilant in your food choices and daily exercise to prevent this from happening or minimize the gain. In addition, symptoms of depression can include loss of appetite and weight loss in some people, while others may have increased appetite, carbohydrate cravings, and weight gain.

Weight gain following antidepressant therapy may indicate recovery in those who had weight loss as a symptom, or it may be related to taking the medication. Weight gain is a relatively widespread problem during acute or long-term treatment with antidepressants and is a common reason people stop taking their medications. Be mindful of this possibility, particularly if you are on medication for the long term.

Significant weight gain related to taking antidepressant medications can affect your overall health and cause physical and emotional discomfort and distress. Many people feel worse about themselves, having low self-esteem and low confidence, when they gain substantial weight. Healthy eating may prevent or reduce the likelihood of becoming overweight or obese while on medications for depression or bipolar disorder.

Those already overweight will have to control their total caloric intake to manage their body weight. This is only part of the picture. Controlling your weight also means increasing physical activity (exercise) and decreasing the amount of time spent sitting around. This is not easy to do, but you can take steps to make it less difficult, as I discuss in the "Physical Exercise" section of this chapter. Remember that different antidepressant medications all have different effects on your metabolism, so you should remain open to trying more than one drug (if necessary) until you find one that you tolerate well.

Metabolic Syndrome

Metabolic syndrome is a physical health condition that is frequently seen in those who have depression, particularly if they take certain antidepressants or antipsychotic medications or have signs of general inflammation confirmed by a blood test. Metabolic syndrome is a cause of obesity, diabetes, and cardiovascular risk. In 2014, C. D. Rethorst and other researchers at the University of Texas at Dallas studied a national health survey and found metabolic syndrome in just over 41 percent of people who have depression.

Metabolic syndrome is made up of five physical signs, called *cardiovascular risk factors*, defined by the American Heart Association (AHA) and the National Heart, Lung, and Blood Institute (NHLBI). You need to have at least three out of five of these risk factors to meet the diagnosis. They are:

> Metabolic syndrome can lead to diabetes and long-term physical health consequences such as heart attack, stroke, kidney failure, and more. You want to avoid it if possible.

- Obesity, more prominent in the abdomen (central obesity), with a waist circumference of 102 centimeters (cm) or greater in men and 88 cm or greater in women
- High triglycerides in the blood: 150 milligrams per deciliter (mg/dL) or higher
- Low HDL cholesterol in the blood (the "good" cholesterol): 40 mg/dL or less in men or 50 mg/dL or less in women
- High blood pressure: 130/85 mm Hg (millimeters of mercury) or greater, or treatment for high blood pressure
- High fasting blood sugar: 100 mg/dL or higher (or being on medication for high blood sugar)

Metabolic syndrome can be initially managed with lifestyle changes. These include getting adequate sleep, engaging in regular cardiovascular exercise with strength training, and following a low carbohydrate diet that includes healthy fats (olive oil, avocados). Sometimes medication is needed to control the elevated blood pressure, cholesterol, or blood sugar. Researchers have also looked at medications to treat the underlying inflammation associated with metabolic syndrome, but further studies are needed.

What Is a Balanced, Nutritious Diet, Anyway?

Since you have control over what you eat, it is in your best interest to nourish your brain in the most beneficial way. To help you improve your eating habits and reach the goal of a healthy, balanced diet, I include basic nutritional information in this section.

A comprehensive and easy-to-use resource to learn about healthy eating is the US Department of Agriculture (USDA) *Dietary Guidelines for Americans 2015–2020*, which can be found online at www.health.gov/dietaryguide lines/2015/guidelines. These are evidence-based nutritional guidelines designed to promote health, reduce the risk of chronic diseases, and reduce overweight and obesity through improved nutrition and physical activity. The guidelines are not specific to depression but address general health and well-being.

The USDA *Dietary Guidelines 2015–2020* describe a healthy diet and lifestyle as one that

- emphasizes more whole or minimally processed foods and plant-based foods in a healthy eating pattern across the lifespan;
- is focused on variety, nutrient density, and the amount of food;
- emphasizes fruits, vegetables, whole grains, and lean protein (lean meats, poultry, fish, beans, eggs, and nuts);
- emphasizes fat-free or low-fat milk and dairy products;
- is low in saturated fats, trans fats, cholesterol, salt (sodium), and added sugars; and
- meets the *Physical Activity Guidelines for Americans* (also available online at www.health.gov/paguidelines/guidelines).

You may have seen these recommendations drawn as a food pyramid in the past. The guidelines now display healthy food as portions divided on a dinner plate, with fruits, vegetables, whole grains, lean protein (such as chicken or fish), and a small amount of dairy (figure 1.2). There is an easy-to-use interactive website to help you understand the food portions at www .choosemyplate.gov.

Visit this website for many helpful tips on healthy eating, including menu choices and specific calorie goals for your age and gender. Optimal daily caloric intake depends on your gender, age, current weight, activity level, and goals for maintaining, losing, or gaining weight. This is individual for each person; your family doctor or a dietitian can help you identify your caloric goal.

The USDA *Dietary Guidelines* (box 1.3) recommend that you make half your plate fruits and vegetables, or that adults eat five one-half cup servings

FIGURE 1.2. **Example of healthy food portions divided on a dinner plate**

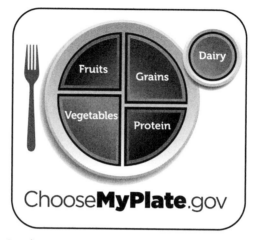

Based on original illustration of the US Department of Agriculture, www.choosemyplate.gov.

of different colored vegetables and three one-half cup servings of whole fruits per day. The recommended portion of protein for adults is approximately one-quarter of your plate at each meal, roughly the size of your palm, or 3 ounces per serving. Grains should be two 3-ounce servings per day for active adults, or approximately one-quarter of your plate at each meal. Half of these should be whole grains (barley, oats, brown rice, quinoa) rather than refined grains (white flour, white rice). Dairy should be low fat and used in moderation, as should other fats—these should preferably come from olive or canola oil, nuts, or avocados. Salt (sodium), often hidden in prepared and baked foods, should be limited to 2,300 milligrams (mg) per day. Many people use spices and herbs in cooking preparation instead of salt to enhance the flavor. You can meet these guidelines by following a healthy US-based diet, a vegetarian diet, or the Mediterranean Diet. The USDA *Dietary Guidelines* website has links to each of these.

Eating for energy and balanced mental health means that you have three small to medium meals per day plus one or two healthy snacks as you choose. Don't skip meals. A snack might be a piece of fruit, or string cheese and a few walnuts or almonds, but no chips, fries, candy, soda, or junk food. Eat real food. You should stay well hydrated by drinking 6 to 8 glasses of water per day. Avoid sugary drinks and diet soda. Avoid alcohol, as it is a depressant and not good for your general physical and mental health. Avoid tobacco and street drugs. Remember, a balanced healthy diet leaves you satisfied and not hungry for more.

BOX 1.3. USDA 2015–2020 Dietary Guidelines for Americans

This list summarizes the key points in maintaining a healthy body and weight.

- Increase whole grains, vegetables, and whole fruits in your diet.

- Eat a variety of vegetables, especially dark green, red, and orange vegetables and legumes (beans, lentils, peas).

- Eat at least half of all grains as whole grains (barley, oats, brown rice, quinoa) instead of refined grains (white flour and white rice).

- Choose a variety of protein foods, which include seafood, lean meat and poultry, eggs, and plant-based proteins like beans, lentils, soy products, nuts, and seeds.

- Use oils in moderation (canola or olive oils, 5 to 6 teaspoons per day), nuts, avocados.

- Reduce or eliminate the amount of sugar-sweetened beverages you drink.

- Focus on the total number of calories consumed. Monitor your food intake.

- Be aware of portion size: choose smaller portions or lower-calorie options.

- Eat less than 10 percent of your calories per day from added sugars (12.5 teaspoons per day).

- Limit daily sodium (salt) intake to less than 2,300 milligrams per day.

- Eat less than 10 percent of calories from saturated fats (butter, cream, cheese, fatty meats) by replacing them with monounsaturated and poly-unsaturated fatty acids (olive oil, canola oil, walnuts, flax seeds, sunflower seeds, fish such as salmon, trout, or mackerel).

- Choose fat-free or low-fat milk and milk products (milk, yogurt, cheese) or soy.

- Use alcohol in moderation.

- Eliminate foods that contain synthetic sources of trans fats, such as partially hydrogenated oils (read the food labels).

- Stay physically active and meet the *Physical Activity Guidelines for Americans*.

Source: US Department of Agriculture and US Department of Health and Human Services, *Dietary Guidelines for Americans 2015–2020*, 8th ed. (Washington, DC: Government Printing Office, 2015), www.health.gov/dietaryguidelines/2015/guidelines.

Pay attention to portion sizes at home and when you eat out, because they have slowly increased in size over the years at restaurants and in the home. For example, a healthy serving of protein such as meat or fish is only 3 ounces, about the size of a deck of cards or your palm. A serving (one-half cup) of fresh fruit is about the size of half a baseball. One cup of cereal (a serving) is the size of your fist. One serving of rice, pasta, or potato is one-half cup, the size of half a baseball. Table 1.4 gives you some sample food serving sizes to help you estimate what you are eating.

TABLE 1.4. Sample Food Serving Sizes: What One Serving Looks Like

GRAIN PRODUCTS
1 cup of cereal flakes = fist
1 pancake = compact disc
½ cup of cooked rice, pasta, or potato = ½ baseball
1 slice of bread = cell phone
1 piece of cornbread = bar of soap

VEGETABLES AND FRUIT
1 cup of salad greens = baseball
1 baked potato = fist
1 med. fruit = baseball
½ cup of fresh fruit = ½ baseball
¼ cup of raisins = large egg

DAIRY
1½ oz. cheese = 4 stacked dice
½ cup of ice cream = ½ baseball

FATS
1 tsp. margarine or spreads = 1 dice

MEAT AND ALTERNATIVES
3 oz. meat, fish, and poultry = deck of cards
3 oz. grilled / baked fish = checkbook
2 Tbsp. peanut butter = ping pong ball

Source: National Institutes of Health and National Heart, Lung, and Blood Institute, "Serving Size Card," accessed October 2017, www.nhlbi.nih.gov/health/educational /wecan/downloads/servingcard7.pdf.

You have to work to build a healthy eating pattern—it does not come naturally to many people. It's hard to make healthy choices when you don't feel well, and eating well is difficult to do when you're depressed. Your appetite may be gone, and when that happens, your interest in food and nutrition is decreased and takes on less importance. Favorite foods or a nice meal may not bring you the same pleasure it once did. You may be so fatigued that grocery shopping and cooking, and even eating, is a major effort. You might feel that healthy foods are too complicated to cook, and you're too tired to do it. Some people complain that healthy foods are more expensive, but that's not necessarily true when you watch portion sizes.

When you're depressed, it's much easier to skip meals or eat fast food, takeout, and prepared foods that are higher in fats and salt and not as healthy for you or your brain. Grocery shopping and cooking may seem overwhelming, but try to remind yourself how important it is for your mental and physical health. You need the nutrients from a healthy diet as fuel for your body and brain to operate at their best.

Healthy eating does not have to be a chore. Choose which nutritious foods you like and balance your preferences. You don't always have to go for the broccoli because you "should." Don't deprive yourself of small portions of your favorite food on occasion. Avoiding your favorites can lead to overeating and a loss of pleasure in life. Eat enough to satisfy your appetite and not more, being mindful of portion sizes as mentioned above.

You may find it easier to stick to a healthy diet when you plan ahead. Do this at times of the day when you have the most energy. First, make a grocery shopping list of healthy foods. There are websites that can help you with easy menu planning. Try to go shopping at times when the store is least crowded and you are not hungry, and if possible, bring a friend along to help you. Many markets have a salad bar with healthy choices to start—just watch the amount of salad dressing you use. Cook soups, stews, or chicken in large batches so that you can freeze portions for later use, on days when fatigue sets in. Buy vegetables and throw them in a crock pot, if you have one, to cook all day—the result is a healthy, nourishing meal with little effort. Cook on days or times of day when you have more energy, or ask a friend or family member to help you do it together. Make your grocery shopping and cooking part of your weekly routine and schedule them in. Some people find that a weekend day is the best time for them to shop and cook for the week. Then just do it even if you don't really feel like it.

Some people experience anxiety along with their depression, and with this they may have unusual food cravings and a tendency to snack on junk food. Try to resist this temptation. Have only healthy foods and snacks at home to reach for when the urge is there. Bring a healthy snack with you to work and have it readily available. A piece of fruit, yogurt, or twelve (yes, twelve) walnuts or almonds are far better choices than chips or candy. Talk to your doctor if unusual food cravings persist. Keep variety in your diet as a way to ensure your body gets the many nutrients it needs. Variety also helps keep you from getting bored with the same old menus. Try a cooking class. This will also get you out of the house and introduce you to new people and new ideas, which are good for your depression.

Eating out at restaurants can also sabotage the best intentions of maintaining a healthy diet and weight. Try to stick to your plan of portion control, limiting fats and salt. Do your best to avoid fast food restaurants. Order an appetizer and salad instead of a main course, request that the salad dressing or sauce be put on the side, share a main course, or ask for a doggie bag to bring the rest of your entrée home for the next day.

If following a healthy diet and regular exercise program does not solve your weight-gain problem, speak with your physician about alternative medications for depression and sleep. Other options include joining a support group plan such as Weight Watchers, getting a referral to the Weight Center at your local hospital, or speaking with your physician about a medication to help counteract the weight-gaining potential of antidepressant medications.

I heard an interesting presentation recently about mindfulness and intentional eating. It was by a nutritionist in Lenox, Massachusetts, named Judy Deutsch. Her point was that we often rush through our meals, sometimes eating while standing up, driving, or in front of the TV. You tend to eat one-third more food this way, by not paying attention. She had these suggestions:

- Be in the moment while eating, paying attention to what you eat, how it tastes, the texture and smell.

- Enjoy every morsel. Use fresh fruits and vegetables; they taste better and cost less.

- Try new things, like new foods or recipes, herbs, or new cooking methods.

- Plan your eating times, food shopping, and food preparation times.

I like her approach!

PHYSICAL EXERCISE

You have often heard that physical exercise is good for your body and overall health. Did you know that it is also good for your brain, that exercise can alleviate depression? Prevention of and improvement in mild to moderate depressive and anxiety symptoms have been found with physical exercise. Because of this strong evidence, exercise has been included in the 2010 *Practice Guideline for the Treatment of Patients with Major Depressive Disorder*, third edition, by the American Psychiatric Association (APA). And in Great Britain, physical exercise is one of the first treatments used for depression.

It used to be thought that the brain was a fixed organ, that we could not grow new brain cells or repair brain cell damage. Scientists have since learned that the brain is constantly being rewired and can grow new nerve cells throughout life.

Another way the brain is stimulated to make new brain cells is with a chemical in our bodies called BDNF (brain-derived neurotrophic factor). BDNF acts like brain fertilizer; it improves the function of neurons, encourages their growth, and protects them. BDNF turns on genes to produce more neurotransmitters, releasing antioxidants and essential proteins. Physical exercise increases BDNF throughout the brain, including the hippocampus, the area of the brain that helps to regulate emotions and memory. So now we see how aerobic exercise, complex physical activity, and learning a new skill all have beneficial effects on the brain.

The benefits of physical exercise as a treatment for depression are that it

- increases a brain chemical called BDNF which promotes the growth of new brain cells
- helps to regulate brain chemicals (*neurotransmitters*)
- helps to keep the level of stress hormones normal, relieving stress
- increases feelings of confidence, self-esteem, competence, and sense of mastery
- has a positive effect on your mood
- improves your sense of well-being
- releases the "feel good" hormones (*endorphins*)
- improves the quality of your sleep, which in turn improves your mood disorder
- helps to overcome the inertia and sedentary lifestyle that often comes with depression
- increases your social contacts (in an exercise class or in neighborhood or health club interactions)

- builds endurance and physical strength, which combats fatigue
- helps manage your weight

Regular physical exercise may be helpful alone or when used in addition to standard antidepressant treatment. This is called an *augmentation strategy*. Exercise is also considered part of a relapse prevention plan (see chapter 7) and may be associated with lower relapse rates. It is also a way for you to take a more active role in managing your depression. Before beginning an exercise program, discuss your plan with your physician. Mention any physical health concerns, such as heart disease or bone or joint problems.

Depression symptoms may make it more difficult to start and stick with an exercise program. These symptoms include loss of interest in activities, decreased physical and mental energy, decreased motivation, and loss of focus and concentration. It's hard to make healthy choices when you don't feel well. Some people believe that they don't have enough time for physical exercise, that they're too tired or embarrassed, that it's boring or won't help, or that other things in life are more important. Don't despair. You can deal with these challenges by trying the effective steps listed in box 1.4.

First, choose an exercise activity that you enjoy, or used to enjoy, and can do regularly. Once you pick your exercise program, sticking with it is the most important part. *How do you do that when you're depressed?* That's a challenge! Make exercise part of your daily routine and schedule it as a key part of your day. Here is where *action precedes motivation*. This means that you should start your exercise program now and keep at it, even if you don't really feel like doing it. The motivation for doing it will come later.

If you have not exercised in a while, start slowly and gradually build up your time and effort. Commit to walking around the block for 10 minutes each day, and then gradually increase the amount of time you walk each

Brain cells, called *neurons*, have a repair and recovery system in response to stress or illness that leads to new cell growth. This is called *neurogenesis*. It is important because we know that with depression, the brain shrinks in size. So the ability to repair and make new brain cells is fundamental in our recovery from a mood disorder. Skills that have to be learned (like playing the piano, learning a new language, responding to stress, or learning a cognitive behavioral therapy skill) challenge the brain to grow and set down new networks of brain cells (*neural networks*).

week. Or start by walking 10 minutes away from your house, and then 10 minutes back home, and gradually increase your time. You may want to purchase an inexpensive step counter, a small plastic device you clip to your waist that counts each step as you go about your daily life. The goal is to add 1,000 steps in the course of your day, so that you eventually walk up to 10,000 steps daily. Set realistic, achievable goals. Incorporate small changes into your daily activities, such as walking more places, taking the stairs instead of the elevator, or getting off the subway or bus two stops earlier.

Sometimes you can get stuck in a pattern with a lot of negative automatic thoughts about physical exercise. Thoughts like "I'm no good at this," "I'm too tired," or "It won't make a difference in me anyway" will get in the way of achieving your goals. One way to address these intrusive thoughts is with the Mood and Thought Monitoring Exercise in chapter 8. Another resource for you to try are the ideas and exercises presented in *The Wellness Workbook for Bipolar Disorder*, by Louisa Grandin Sylvia, PhD.

Exercise Guidelines

What counts as exercise? Exercise is any physical activity or movement of the body that uses energy. The American College of Sports Medicine considers a regular exercise program to be essential for most adults. It endorses one that includes cardiorespiratory, resistance, flexibility, and neuromotor exercise training, beyond the usual activities of daily living, to improve and maintain physical fitness and health.

A sedentary lifestyle, defined as having limited physical activity, is associated with many chronic illnesses such as obesity, diabetes, heart disease, metabolic syndrome, osteoporosis, and others. Aerobic exercise and resistance, or strength, training can help to reverse some of the degenerative processes common in chronic illnesses and decrease the risk of these diseases. Amazing people have shown us that it is still possible to get physical exercise even if you have a limiting physical disability; you just have to be creative and perhaps get some help in getting started.

Muscle burns more calories than does fat or bone, and adding muscle by strength training increases the energy you use daily. You also burn more calories for 72 hours after a strength-training workout. Resistance training decreases the belly fat commonly seen in older men and women and in metabolic syndrome; increases physical functioning; decreases the chance of getting type 2 diabetes; decreases resting blood pressure; increases bone density; decreases fatigue, anxiety, and depression; and increases cognitive abilities and self-esteem.

BOX 1.4. Get Started with Exercise and Keep It Going

- Do what you enjoy or used to enjoy. Do something that is fun.

- Assess what type of exercise resources are available to you. Look for a safe area to walk in your neighborhood. Find out if there is a community center or health club facility available to you with exercise classes or equipment. Consider whether you have or can invest in home exercise equipment. See what kind of social supports are available to keep you motivated to exercise.

- Plan a specific and realistic activity that you can do. Define the type of activity, how often you will do it, and for how long (frequency and duration).

- Make exercise a priority in your day and a key part of your daily routine.

- Believe that the exercise will benefit you—this will make it easier to do.

- List the pros and cons of exercising compared to having a sedentary lifestyle.

- Come up with your own personal reasons for exercising.

- Exercise with a partner (a walking partner or people in a class)—you will have to be accountable to him or her to show up and exercise together. This is a good social support.

- Consider having a personal trainer help you set up a program, then monitor and motivate you.

- Identify and address any barriers ahead of time, such as the time of day, your energy level, balancing other obligations, too busy, too tired, too sick, bored, embarrassed, and so forth.

- Work toward a goal that has personal meaning. This could be a walking or running distance or length of time, or a specific exercise accomplishment.

- Train for a charity event (such as a walk-, run-, or bike-a-thon).

- Track your progress in a journal or log and review it periodically.

- Focus on the activity and not on your performance. Try not to make comparisons to your past or others' performance.

- As you get stronger, vary your activity so that you avoid boredom and repetitive injury.

- Give yourself credit for what you can do now.

It is recommended that you do a combination of

aerobic activities that increase your heart rate and breathing (see the examples in table 1.7),
strength activities that build and maintain bones and muscle, and
balance and stretching activities that increase physical stability and flexibility, such as yoga, tai chi, or just basic stretches.

When you do aerobic exercise, your body's large muscles (such as your quadriceps or hamstring muscles in your legs) move for a sustained period, your heart rate and breathing rate increase, and you get sweaty.

There are three components of aerobic exercise that influence the amount of benefit you get from each workout: intensity, frequency, and duration (table 1.5). So, for example, you might work out for 30 minutes per session (duration) three times per week (frequency) with moderate effort (intensity).

Strength activities are those that cause the body's muscles to work against a force, such as when you pick up a weight or press against a resistance band. This is also called resistance exercise. Building muscle keeps your body strong and helps you burn more calories. Muscle-strengthening activities also have three components that influence the amount of benefit you derive from the exercise: intensity, repetitions, and frequency (table 1.6). You might lift 20 pounds of weight (intensity) 15 times (repetitions) during three sessions per week (frequency). Examples of aerobic exercise are found in table 1.7.

TABLE 1.5. **Components of Aerobic Exercise**

COMPONENTS OF AEROBIC EXERCISE	WHAT IT MEANS	HOW IT'S DEFINED
Intensity	How hard you work, how much effort	Mild, moderate, or vigorous activity
Frequency	How often you do the activity	Number of times per day or week
Duration	How long you do the activity	Length of time in minutes

TABLE 1.6. Components of Resistance Exercise

COMPONENTS OF RESISTANCE EXERCISE	WHAT IT MEANS	HOW IT'S DEFINED
Intensity	How much weight you lift, or which color-coded resistance band you use	Weight in pounds or kilograms, or color of band
Repetitions	How many times you lift the weight or repeat the motion	Number of times you repeat the motion (repetitions)
Frequency	How often you do the activity	Number of times per day or week

TABLE 1.7. Examples of Aerobic Exercise Intensity

MODERATE INTENSITY ACTIVITY	VIGOROUS INTENSITY ACTIVITY
• Walking (3.5 mph) • Water aerobics • Biking on level ground • Playing tennis—doubles • Mowing the lawn • Cleaning the house • Dancing • Canoeing, kayaking • Golfing • Gardening • Playing baseball or softball • Playing with children	• Walking fast (4 to 4.5 mph) • Jogging or running (5.0 mph or faster) • Swimming laps • Taking an aerobics or spinning class • Using aerobic equipment (elliptical trainer, etc.) • Biking fast or up hills • Playing tennis—singles • Playing basketball • Playing soccer • Heavy gardening • Hiking uphill • Jumping rope

Sources: US Department of Health and Human Services, *Physical Activity Guidelines for Americans*, HHS, 2008, www.health.gov/paguidelines/guidelines; US Centers for Disease Control and Prevention, "Measuring Physical Activity Intensity," accessed October 2017, www.cdc.gov/physicalactivity/everyone/measuring.

Intensity and Duration of Physical Activity

The recommended exercise guidelines for healthy adults are

- at least 30 minutes of moderate activity 5 times a week and 2 or more days of strength training each week

or

- at least 25 minutes of vigorous activity 3 times a week and 2 or more days of strength training each week

What is considered *moderate or vigorous activity*? Table 1.7 lists examples of both moderate and vigorous activities. The intensity depends on how much effort you are putting into it. To estimate the intensity of your physical activity, use the Talking Test. If you are able to talk while exercising, that is a *moderate* activity. If you are out of breath, that is a *vigorous* activity.

Or you could count your heart rate during exercise to determine whether you are exercising at a moderate or vigorous intensity. Do this by placing two fingers on the side of your neck or on the inside of your wrist and count the heart beats for one minute. Take this number and compare it to the percentage of your target heart rate (HR).

- Your target heart rate is 220 minus your age.
- Exercising at 50 to 60 percent of your target HR is moderate intensity exercise.
- Exercising at 70 to 85 percent of your target HR is vigorous intensity exercise.

Fitness Trends

Some of the trends in physical activity you might find helpful include *high-intensity interval training, circuit training, group training,* and the use of *fitness apps* on your smartphone or tablet. These are generally more effective ways to get a good workout and to stay motivated.

High-intensity interval training is an aerobic activity in which you exercise at your maximum effort for 1 to 2 minutes, then lessen your effort for a minute and repeat this in cycles for a total of 30 minutes. You can do this when walking, running, bicycling, swimming laps, or on an elliptical trainer. For example, when outside you can use a timer or just run or walk as fast as you can from your starting point to the next tree or telephone pole, slow down, then start again.

Circuit training means alternating strength-training exercises for 2 to 3 minutes with 2 minutes of exercise on a treadmill or stationary bike. It's usually done in a gym because the equipment is nearby. There is a popular program on YouTube called *CrossFit*, but it is intense and not for beginners. Other circuit-training programs are *P90X*, workouts based on muscle confusion, and *The Magic Pill*, a 21-day exercise podcast from National Public Radio (on station WBUR).

Group training has become popular in recent years and is both fun and motivational. The term refers to an exercise effort you do together with

> Train your body and your mind will follow.

other people, like running up the stairs in a football stadium or running a distance through your city or town. Projects such as Fitness Tribes and the November Project are common examples that you can read about on the internet.

Smartphones (and tablets) have many fitness apps that you can subscribe to for free. They help you stay organized, effective, and motivated in your workout. You might want to check out the following apps: Map My Run, Map My Ride, Full Fitness, or Zombies, Run! The following quick and easy apps can easily fit into your workday:

- 1 Minute Desk Workout
- Office Exercise & Stretch Pro
- Headspace
- Barre3
- Seven
- Sworkit

You can see a good overview of these in a *Wall Street Journal* article, "Workouts for the Overworked" (August 29, 2014) at www.wsj.com/articles /fitness-apps-for-exercising-in-15-minutes-or-less-1409353121.

Track Your Progress

As you keep up your exercise program, your strength, endurance, and energy level will improve. The more you do, the stronger you will become, and the more likely you will do the activity. The best advice I have read is to get fit and continue to challenge yourself, raising the bar periodically. The more fit you are physically, the more resilient your brain will become and the better it will function.

Tracking your progress is a good way to monitor your activities, adjust your exercise as you improve, and keep up your motivation. One way to do this is to record the type and duration of your physical activities in a weekly agenda or exercise log. The method you choose is based on personal preference. There are many electronic gadgets for this purpose, some of them wearable, such as a pedometer or the Fitbit among others. Another method is to use the USDA's online tool, SuperTracker (www.choosemyplate.gov /tools-supertracker), which offers a way to track your exercise and your calories over time. The specific tracking method does not matter—the most effective one for you is the one you'll use.

ROUTINE AND STRUCTURE

Routine and consistency in daily life help make your life more manageable and in control. It is thought that small changes in one's daily routine place stress on the body's ability to maintain stability, and that those with mood disorders have a more difficult time adapting to these changes in routine. Paying close attention to daily routines, and to the positive and negative events that influence those routines and cause you stress, increases your stability. This is the basis of social rhythm therapy, a treatment for bipolar disorder, which has some benefit to mood disorders in general.

Many people with depression have a difficult time going about their daily activities. Endless hours of empty time alone is not healthy for anyone, however, and will only worsen your symptoms. So it is essential to maintain a regular routine and structure to each day, even when you don't feel like it. Schedule your time and try to follow that schedule, but also be flexible with yourself. Keep your schedule in an agenda or appointment book (paper or electronic) that you carry with you. Having a daily structure and following a routine will also help you better manage the lack of interest and decreased energy that often come with depression.

Plan your time each day to include a *balance* of these things:

- Responsibilities and obligations: things you do at work, home, school, with family.
- Daily self-care:
  - meals and nutrition
  - medications, treatments, therapy
  - personal care: showering, shaving, brushing your teeth, getting dressed
  - sleep
  - exercise
- Social contacts—being with people you like has a positive effect on your mood:
  - keep regular contact with safe people and situations
  - avoid isolation

- Positive experiences:
  - pleasant and pleasurable activities: it is not enough to eliminate the negative experiences in life—you also need to include positive and pleasurable experiences
  - mastery of activities: activities that are somewhat difficult for you to do and are a challenge give a sense of being competent and effective—learning a new skill or overcoming an obstacle is one way to achieve mastery
  - purpose in life: include activities that give you a sense of purpose

Keep your daily schedule

- Prioritized: understand what is most important for you to do.
- Measurable: put a time frame around each activity (instead of open-ended time).
- Attainable and realistic: start with the things that you can do *now*, in your current state:
  - pace yourself
  - break large complex tasks down into small steps that are more realistic and manageable
  - don't overschedule—this creates more stress and the potential for failure
  - learn to set limits and say no when you are overextended
- Concrete and specific: clearly define each goal and task.
- Flexible: understand where you are and what you can do at any given time and modify your schedule as needed. Do not compare your current self and abilities to past levels of performance or functioning.

Keep a list of activities, exercise, and people you enjoy (table 1.8) to make it easier to include them in your daily structure.

TABLE 1.8. **Activities, Exercise, and People You Enjoy**

Things I like (or used to like) to do:

Types of physical exercise I like (or used to like)—only those things I can do now:

People I like to keep in contact with:

AVOID ISOLATION

Social interaction is important for all of us, particularly when faced with an illness like a mood disorder. It provides many benefits, such as a feeling of acceptance, increased self-esteem, a chance for friendship and fun, and access to someone who can provide support if you need it. We all need to have social contact and support to maintain our emotional well-being and protect against major depression.

With depression, there is a tendency to withdraw from the activities of your daily life and to avoid contact with friends and family. You may prefer to stay at home, not get dressed or answer the telephone, and just do nothing. Getting in touch with others or responding to those who are trying to help you is often quite difficult. Symptoms of depression such as fatigue and lack of interest may contribute to your withdrawal. This type of alone time is often lonely, closed off, and adds to your sense of sadness. Resist the urge to isolate and withdraw from your life. Isolation is not healthy for you or your brain. Social isolation and lack of social support increase the risk of developing depression and may prolong episodes of depression.

Examples of isolation and withdrawal include:

- Staying alone at home most of the time, without others around
- Avoiding conversations with your family or friends, in person or by not making or returning telephone calls
- Not going out to be with other people
- Skipping your usual errands and human interactions
- Avoiding activities you once enjoyed
- Canceling plans with others for no particular reason
- Not making new plans
- Canceling doctor's appointments

Isolation versus Solitude

All alone time is not the same. Spending *some* time alone each day, without feeling lonely, can be beneficial. Solitude, rather than isolation, has a purpose and provides a sense of contentment and enjoyment. It allows you to think, self-reflect, and relax or replenish yourself when overwhelmed. Solitude is something you choose to experience, in contrast to the isolation of depression. Everyone needs a bit of alone time in their lives. A quiet walk outdoors, reading, or working on a favorite hobby are examples of solitude that can be valuable to your well-being. Even though solitude is alone time, it is not the same as the isolation and withdrawal that comes with depression.

People vary in how much they value and feel comfortable being alone. That is built into your disposition, the way you were born, and each person is different. You have to know yourself and your personal preferences. For example, farmers tending to their cattle or crops all day or fishermen at sea may feel quite content and not lonely or isolated, even though they do not see other people for days at a time. They are not bothered by being alone in their chosen place. This may be a healthy decision for them. Another person may not feel the same way and need to be surrounded by others, such as by living in a large city. People choose lifestyles with varying degrees of solitude, based on what is healthy for them.

How do you *avoid isolation and withdrawal*? The first step is to recognize when it is happening. If you notice yourself spending more time alone, not by choice but because you are fatigued and have no interest or energy, this is isolation. If you find yourself avoiding people and activities for no particular reason, this is withdrawal. Know the signs of isolation for you and include these on your Action Plan for Relapse Prevention (see chapter 7).

Once you have identified your alone time as isolation and withdrawal, take steps to prevent it. Avoiding isolation when depressed can be a challenge. Do not wait until you "feel like it" to get out and be with others. Push yourself a little and just do it, a bit at a time. Make a point of returning telephone calls from friends and family who are helpful and positive. Don't substitute text messaging for real-time phone calls and face-to-face contact with others. Set your expectations to do the activities you can do now and modify them as needed. It can be overwhelming to do everything you managed when well, so break your activities down into small steps. Get out of the house. Do one or two errands at a time, not a dozen. Say hello to the store clerk. For now, walk for 10 minutes around the block rather than tackling your usual exercise routine. Eventually, it will all become easier to do.

A written routine and schedule can help you manage the tendency to withdraw (table 1.9). You can do this on paper or an electronic device. That way, you have something concrete to follow for the times when you are tempted to isolate. The key is to stick to your schedule even when you don't feel like it. Hold yourself accountable for following through. Then give yourself credit for this accomplishment.

TABLE 1.9. Daily Schedule

DATE	MONDAY	TUESDAY	WEDNESDAY
awake @			
7			
8			
9			
10			
11			
12			
1			
2			
3			
4			
5			
6			
7			
8			
9			
bedtime @			

THURSDAY	FRIDAY	SATURDAY	SUNDAY

Mood Disorders

Sometimes we experience a combination of physical, emotional, and interpersonal symptoms for such a long time that we don't even recognize them as symptoms. We get used to them and think they are normal.
—MARJORIE HANSEN SHAEVITZ

A *mood disorder* is a type of psychiatric illness that includes major depression and bipolar disorder. These are biologically based, treatable conditions of the brain that involve a disturbance in our mood or state of mind, the part of our inner self that colors and drives our thoughts, feelings, and behaviors. The two conditions are grouped together because they share some of the same clinical characteristics.

MAJOR DEPRESSION

Major depression, also called *depression*, *major depressive disorder*, or *unipolar depression*, affects your thoughts, feelings, behaviors, relationships, activities, interests, and many other aspects of life. Someone who has depression often has trouble functioning in the ordinary activities of daily living. Depression is most often a *relapsing and remitting* yet treatable illness. A relapsing and remitting condition means that the symptoms come and go, in varying intervals of time called *episodes*. An episode of depression may last weeks, months, or longer. It may differ in how deep or severe it is. Many people have repeat episodes over time and feel well in between—the pattern is unique to each person. Some have one or a few episodes and then none for many years. It's nearly impossible to predict the duration of each episode and to know exactly if or when a person may have future episodes.

This may come as potentially discouraging news to those who are expecting an immediate "cure" to their mood disorder and never have a return of symptoms. Unfortunately, for many people, this is not the case. While you might have long periods, years or decades, of feeling well, there is a

Researchers have observed that approximately 60 percent of those who have one episode of depression will have a second at some point in their lives. Seventy percent of those who experience two episodes will have a third, and 90 percent of those who experience three episodes will have a fourth. This is not meant to discourage you, only to help reinforce the importance of seeking treatment and managing your illness.

pretty good chance that another episode will appear at some point in your life. Realistically, depression is a medical condition characterized by ups and downs in your mood over time, more significant but not unlike those *without* a mood disorder who have bad stretches every once in a while. The goal is to keep these repeat episodes mild and to a minimum. This is possible if you take steps to manage your illness daily and respond to your warning signs if they appear. You can also help yourself by strengthening your *resilience skills*, the ways we bounce back from adversity and difficult events in life (like a mental health episode). There is more on resilience in my book *When Someone You Know Has Depression: Words to Say and Things to Do*.

One way to see patterns in your illness and its relationship to life events is to track your daily symptoms on a Mood Chart (table 2.4). This chart is pretty easy to use. All you need to do is make a best-guess estimate of your mood for that day and check the corresponding box on the chart. Then write in the notes section anything that you think may have affected your mood— for example, a change in medication, a stressor or illness, hormonal shifts such as menstruation, the birth of a baby, or menopause.

Tracking these details is a good way to follow your progress and response to treatment. This information can then be used in making treatment decisions with your physician or as a point of discussion in psychotherapy sessions.

One long-held theory of depression is that it involves an imbalance of chemicals in the brain, called *neurotransmitters*. These chemicals help the brain cells (called *neurons*) communicate with each other. Neurotransmitters are found throughout the brain, including in the part that regulates your emotions and behavior. The chemical imbalance may happen when certain life experiences occur in a susceptible person. What makes a person susceptible is not fully understood.

A newer theory of depression is that the interaction of your genes with events in your life (your environment) shapes the complex network of cells in your brain. This is called the *gene × environment* theory. Our *environment* includes the people, thoughts, and events that occur around us, both inside and outside our bodies. This could be inside or outside stress, an illness, or a traumatic event. Examples of stressful life events include a major loss or death, marriage or divorce, a new job or loss of a job, chronic stress, hormonal changes (such as during perimenopause or postpartum), medical illness, substance abuse, sleep disorders, and positive events like the birth of a baby or moving to a new home.

A *gene* is a precise arrangement of molecules (a sequence of DNA) that makes up the chromosomes in our cells. Genes are inherited from each of our parents. They direct the body to make certain proteins that control our normal bodily functions, including those of our brain. Scientists have found genes associated with some disease conditions, such as Huntington disease, cystic fibrosis, and some psychiatric illnesses such as schizophrenia, bipolar disorder, and depression. A recent study by Hyde, Perlis, and associates identified fifteen genes linked to major depression in persons of European descent. And approximately eleven genes associated with a susceptibility to bipolar disorder have been identified. These findings may help us to better understand these illnesses and to design new treatments.

The *gene × environment* theory of depression is thought to work in this way. The brain is sensitive to stressful and traumatic events during vulnerable periods in life. Negative stimulation, such as stress or illness, changes the action of certain genes. When this happens, it affects the shape of the network of cells in our brain (the *neural network*) and its functioning. If stress or illness changes gene activity during a vulnerable period, the genes and our brains do not work as well. In summary, negative stimulation such as stress or illness changes gene activity, which results in dysfunction of the neural network in our brains. If that happens during a vulnerable period, it affects our feelings, thoughts, and behaviors, and the result is depression. Depression is not entirely genetic and not entirely related to life experiences. It requires the "perfect storm" of both coming together at a time when the person is vulnerable.

You may have genetic factors that make you more likely to suffer from depression, but this does not guarantee that you will have the illness. If you are genetically prone to depression, you may not have an episode unless you also experience certain stressful life events. These experiences are thought to affect the genes that regulate your brain functioning.

Depression often runs in families, which supports the idea of a genetic basis for the illness. This was seen in research studies of depression in twins, who by definition share some of the same genetic material. The research showed that first-degree relatives of those who have major depression have an increased risk of depression. This is in part due to shared genes and is separate from shared family experiences. These results provide support for the inherited (genetic) theory of depression.

Major depression is characterized by feeling sad or depressed with loss of interest in activities. The symptoms of depression are psychological, behavioral, and physical. According to the current edition of the standard diagnostic manual of psychiatric disorders from the American Psychiatric Association (the *DSM-5*), to be diagnosed with major depression, you must have at least five of the symptoms listed in box 2.1, lasting for two weeks or more (at least one of the symptoms must be persistent sadness or loss of interest).

People can have various combinations of these nine *DSM-5* criteria for depression, which creates different subtypes of depression (e.g., *atypical, psychotic, melancholic,* or *seasonal*). For an in-depth discussion of these symptoms of depression, see Aaron Beck and Brad Alford's *Depression: Causes and Treatment.* There are also many reliable online resources from the National Institute of Mental Health (NIMH) and the Depression and Bipolar Support Association (DBSA).

What does an episode of depression *feel like?* Living with it is very hard on you and your family and friends. Depression is not just "feeling blue" for a day. It is far beyond sadness. With depression comes deep despair, physical and emotional pain, and suffering. There is often a near paralysis, being unable to participate in and enjoy life, physically and mentally. The hours and days seem endless, full of anguish and misery. With depression, the world is gray and murky, and you see only the negative side of life. You may feel guilty, worthless, and without hope. Irritability may be your main

---

BOX 2.1. **Criteria for Depression**

- sad, depressed, or irritable feelings most of the day
- loss of interest or pleasure in most activities
- sleep changes—too much, too little, or with early morning awakening
- weight loss or gain (without trying)

- loss of energy
- decreased ability to think or concentrate
- restlessness or the sensation of being physically slowed down
- thoughts of worthlessness, hopelessness, guilt
- thoughts of death and suicide

Source: American Psychiatric Association, *Diagnostic and Statistical Manual of Mental Disorders,* 5th ed. (Washington, DC: APA, 2013).

response to the world around you. You lose interest in the things you used to like and may not experience any pleasure. Motivation is nearly gone. Sleep may not come, or there may be too much of it, yet it is hard to get out of bed and move about. Fatigue is overwhelming. Food has no taste. You withdraw from people and activities and may lose friends. Communication and small talk is a major effort. Your thinking slows down, and it is hard to concentrate and focus. School and work suffer. Projects, assignments, and the mail pile up, and you may spend hours just staring, unable to approach the task at hand. The thoughts you have are often distorted and negative, yet they seem quite believable to you. Your thinking may be quite disorganized. And at times, you may believe that death will bring relief.

BIPOLAR DISORDER

Bipolar disorder, which used to be called manic-depressive disorder, is a related brain illness that causes marked fluctuations in your mood. Like major depression, it is a lifelong relapsing and remitting mood disorder that significantly affects daily life and is thought to be caused by a dysfunction in the network of neurons in the brain. Symptoms of bipolar disorder typically appear in the late teens or early adulthood, although some people have their first symptoms in childhood. Bipolar disorder is characterized by periodic intense emotional states called *episodes*, with extreme elevated mood or irritability (*mania* or *hypomania*) alternating with periodic episodes of depression. These episodes come in cycles, in a different pattern for each person. In bipolar disorder, many people spend more of their illness time in the depressed phase rather than the elevated (manic) phase of the disorder. Often, a person experiences depression symptoms first and mania/hypomania symptoms some time later.

The symptoms of bipolar depression are very similar to those of major depression and may make it initially difficult to tell the difference between the two.

To be diagnosed with bipolar disorder, according to the *DSM-5*,

a person must be currently experiencing his or her first manic/
hypomanic episode

or

be known to have had a manic/hypomanic episode at some time in the
past.

The *DSM-5* also states that to be diagnosed with a manic episode, you need to have experienced an elevated or irritable mood that impairs your functioning for at least one week as well as three or more of the symptoms listed in box 2.2.

Different types of bipolar disorder span a spectrum of these symptoms, called *bipolar I, bipolar II, bipolar spectrum*, and *mixed states*. The type depends on the intensity and duration of the elevated mood symptoms. A person who has bipolar I usually has manic episodes and depressive episodes, and may spend about 30 percent of his time in a depressed state and 10 percent in a manic state. Someone who has bipolar II has hypomanic episodes and prolonged depressive episodes, specifically, with about 50 percent of her time in a depressed state and 1 percent in a manic or hypomanic state. The symptoms of bipolar spectrum fall in between. A manic episode is one of elevated mood or irritability, hypomanic episodes are similar but shorter and less intense, and mixed episodes are a combination of depression and mania or hypomania that occur at the same time. There is also a type of bipolar disorder characterized by a pattern of rapidly changing back and forth between mania and depression, with four or more episodes in the course of one year. This is called *rapid cycling*.

What does bipolar disorder *feel like*? Living through the different phases of depressed, manic, hypomanic, or mixed episodes is very hard. When depressed, you may withdraw from friends and family or feel too irritable to be with people. You may often be unable to concentrate and function well at work or school. As in major depression, the days are long and endless. Being manic or hypomanic is like having a storm inside your head. Your thoughts and speech race from topic to topic without completing a thought. You may

---

BOX 2.2. Criteria of Mania

- inflated sense of self or grandiosity

- increased goal-directed activity or psychomotor agitation (purposeless activity)

- decreased need for sleep

- racing thoughts

- distractibility, poor concentration

- pressured speech, which is a certain way of being more talkative than usual

- high-risk behavior (such as excessive spending, impulsive sexual behavior, and so on)

Source: American Psychiatric Association, *Diagnostic and Statistical Manual of Mental Disorders*, 5th ed. (Washington, DC: APA, 2013).

be too disorganized and distracted to function well without realizing it at the time. In fact, when manic, you might think that you can do anything you choose, and that you have great ideas. You may start and stop multiple projects without finishing any of them. You feel a minimal need for sleep, yet you feel energized, not tired. You may have extreme impulses and may engage in high-risk activities, such as exorbitant shopping, excessive sexual behaviors, or driving too fast. Your impulses may lead to making poor financial or business decisions. All of this has an effect on your life and your relationships with friends, family, and work colleagues.

MAKING THE DIAGNOSIS OF A MOOD DISORDER

There are no blood tests for mood disorders and no scans readily available outside a research setting. An illness of the brain leads to changes in the chemicals, cells, and structure of the brain that until recently have been difficult to observe and measure. This difficulty has meant that people have a hard time believing the disorders were real, adding to the stigma of mental illness.

Brain imaging techniques are now used in research, including magnetic resonance imaging (MRI), positron emission tomography (PET), and functional magnetic resonance imaging (fMRI). Early evidence from these scans suggests that the brains of people with mood disorders may differ from the brains of healthy people. For example, scientists have learned that in bipolar disorder, genetic differences affect the production and release of chemicals between brain cells. This shapes how the brain works, leading to changes in our thoughts, feelings, and behaviors. In another study, researchers at the University of North Carolina School of Medicine reported on a technique using a *resting-state functional brain connectivity MRI (rs-fcMRI)* scan to predict therapeutic responses to talk therapy in those who have major depression.

In clinical practice, to make the diagnosis, your doctor will take your vital signs (heart rate, blood pressure), do a basic physical exam, and ask you a detailed series of questions about how you are feeling and what kind of symptoms you are having. Topics include your sleep, appetite, weight, interests, daily activities, work or school, social supports, and thoughts of harming yourself. Testing your ability to think, reason, express yourself and remember, and observing your mood, behavior, and general appearance, called a *mental health assessment*, is the next step in diagnosing a mental illness. You will also be asked about your family's medical history. Next blood and urine tests will be done to make sure that no other physical problem is causing your illness, such as a thyroid condition or street drugs in your system (these would appear on a toxicology screen).

Treatment-Resistant Depression

Choosing a treatment plan for depression is a complex medical decision requiring an experienced psychiatrist. In reality, however, many people receive their initial treatment from their family doctor or primary care physician (PCP). This is often done in consultation with a psychiatrist to determine the best choice of antidepressant medication. Even in the best hands, some people don't see an improvement in their symptoms or level of functioning after one course of treatment. They may get discouraged, stating, "Those antidepressants don't work for me!" Until recently, it was thought that perhaps such individuals were just not receiving an adequate dose of medication, were not taking it as prescribed, or were not tolerating it because of side effects. Psychiatrists now have a better understanding of those who appear to be treatment resistant.

First, it's helpful to understand the language when thinking about this topic (table 2.1).

TABLE 2.1. **Definitions of Antidepressant Treatment Responses**

Response	Partial improvement in symptoms and at least a 50% reduction in depression severity as measured by standardized rating questionnaires
Remission	Depressive symptoms completely cleared
Relapse	Return of full depressive symptoms after *partial* recovery from an episode
Recurrence	Return of full depressive symptoms following *full* recovery from an episode

Source: Adapted from A. A. Nierenberg and L. M. DeCecco, "Definitions of Antidepressant Treatment Response, Remission, Nonresponse, Partial Response, and Other Relevant Outcomes: A Focus on Treatment-Resistant Depression," *Journal of Clinical Psychiatry* 62, suppl 16 (2001): 15–19.

Response to antidepressant treatment often takes weeks or months. Many people require multiple attempts at treatment to reach a satisfactory response or recovery. Research psychiatrists have learned that antidepressant medications are helpful in 60 to 70 percent of people. About half of those who have depression respond to a first course of antidepressant treatment. Only one-third achieve full remission after a complete course of treatment. About 30 percent of those who have major depression fail to respond to antidepressant medications or psychotherapy and are referred to as *treatment resistant*. This can be quite frustrating. There is no accepted definition of the term *treatment-resistant depression*. It may mean failure to improve after one course of antidepressant with adequate dose and duration, or it may mean failure to respond to three or more courses of antidepressant and other treatments, including talk therapy or electroconvulsive (ECT) therapy over several months. Psychiatrists urge people who have depression not to despair or give up on treatment because it is so difficult to know what will be effective or in whom.

There are three main reasons why antidepressants don't seem to work for some people.

1. Drug selection and dosing issues

First, it's helpful to understand that antidepressants are most effective when given at a certain dose for a particular length of time. But there is no absolutely "correct" dose of medication for all people, because the dose can vary with people's age, gender, weight, physical health, and other medications they are taking. Some people have problems tolerating an antidepressant, and others are genetically predisposed to metabolize the drug at a faster or slower rate. There are many different types of antidepressants, some of which may work better for different symptoms of depression than others.

Treatment failure may occur because the person was not on the most effective choice of antidepressant drug for him. He may have been on too low a dose, or for too short a period of time; or he may have had intolerable side effects that prevented him from reaching his optimal dose. This has become less common in recent years with the introduction of new medications. Drug selection and dosing issues may occasionally happen as nonpsychiatrists, such as PCPs, commonly prescribe antidepressant medications. These providers, while knowledgeable, may not be as familiar with the finer details of these complex drugs, because antidepressants are not necessarily in their area of specialty. Another factor in whether a treatment works is that sometimes, people who have depression have difficulty sticking with a medication and end up skipping doses. This could result from the inconvenience of taking several pills per day, side effects caused by the drug, or other individual reasons.

2. Inaccurate diagnosis

A diagnosis can be inaccurate if, for example, a person who has bipolar disorder seeks help with symptoms that look quite similar to unipolar (major) depression. It can be tricky to tell the difference. If this is her first episode, she may have never had or been observed to have a manic or hypomanic episode, so the diagnosis of bipolar disorder is yet to be made. Unfortunately, someone who has bipolar disorder will not respond well to standard antidepressant therapy and may be incorrectly labeled as being a "treatment failure" or "treatment resistant." Another example is that of people who have various combinations of the nine *DSM-5* criteria for depression. Sometimes the person may have a subtype (atypical, psychotic, melancholic, seasonal) that is not accurately appreciated by the treating provider. Different subtypes of depression are thought to respond differently to the various antidepressant medications. This matters because it can affect the correct selection of antidepressant medication and eventual outcome.

3. Appropriate treatment type, dose, and duration yet still no response

A much smaller group of people do not respond to treatment even with the appropriate type, dose, and duration. They may be experiencing true treatment resistance. Several therapeutic options are available for this category of treatment-resistant depression. Medication options can be to (1) switch to another antidepressant, (2) add a non-antidepressant drug to enhance the effects of the antidepressant (called *augmentation*), or (3) combine different types of antidepressant medications together.

Augmentation strategies include the use of lithium, atypical antipsychotics, thyroid hormone, herbal products, and some newer anticonvulsants. Ketamine is not an antidepressant drug, for example, but it has antidepressant effects in certain individuals. It has a long history as a medication used in anesthesia in higher doses, but it also has the potential for abuse as a "club drug" known as Special K. Ketamine is called an *NMDA glutamate receptor*. The antidepressant effects are thought to be caused by one of the chemical byproducts formed when the body breaks ketamine down into smaller molecules. At low doses, this drug has improved depressive symptoms within 24 hours, but its effects wear off, so it must be given again as an intravenous (IV) infusion (in the veins) or as a mist that you inhale through the nose. Some concern remains because of the limited evidence of its long-term effectiveness, a need for repeated dosages to maintain response, a potential for abuse, and reports of cognitive impairment (difficulty thinking) and bladder problems following repeated use. Ketamine should be reserved for those who have not responded to adequate trials of standard antidepressant treatment; more research is necessary.

Other treatment options for treatment-resistant depression include talk therapy (psychotherapy) and *neurostimulation*, a method that uses very low electrical or magnetic current to stimulate the brain's mood centers.

Neurostimulation can be either a noninvasive or invasive procedure. Available noninvasive methods are *electroconvulsive therapy* (ECT), also called shock therapy, and *repetitive transcranial magnetic stimulation* (rTMS). ECT remains the treatment of choice for most severe, incapacitating forms of depression and for the elderly or those who cannot tolerate antidepressant medications. ECT is performed while using a very short-lasting sedative medication to put you to sleep for a few minutes. Sticky pads are then attached to your scalp to transmit a low electrical current through the scalp to your brain for a few seconds. It does not hurt. ECT is done three times per week for perhaps 12 doses, then on a maintenance schedule as needed. You might have a mild headache and forgetfulness on the day of the procedure.

The other form of noninvasive neurostimulation, rTMS, is done while you are awake and is not painful. It involves transmitting a magnetic current through the scalp to the mood center of your brain using a small wand held to the scalp; rTMS is done daily, 15 minutes at a time, for 6 weeks, then on a maintenance schedule.

Invasive therapies such as deep brain stimulation and vagus nerve stimulation (VNS) require surgery and are not considered lightly. Deep brain stimulation is a surgical procedure in which microelectrodes are carefully placed deep in a very specific area of the brain. Then a tiny electrical current is applied. Deep brain stimulation is generally found to relieve a person's depression. VNS involves the surgical placement of a wire coil that wraps around the vagus nerve in the left side of your neck. The wire is attached to a pulse generator, similar to a heart pacemaker battery, in the left chest wall. The battery sends small electrical signals along the wire coil, which then stimulates the vagus nerve where it interacts with the mood centers of your brain. The pulse generator is usually programmed using a small wand attached to a computer; it sends an electrical signal to the vagus nerve for 20 to 30 seconds every 5 minutes. A person might experience temporary hoarseness during the stimulation.

If you are interested in reading more about people who have the different types of treatment-resistant depression, there is an interesting book called *Still Down: What to Do When Antidepressants Fail*, written by Dean F. MacKinnon. The book uses nine different patient stories, one per chapter, to illustrate the reasons for treatment failure, with a summary and case notes to explain decision points in detail.

Depression in Women

Some women experience depression symptoms that fluctuate as *estrogen* and *progesterone*, the female reproductive hormones produced in the ovaries, normally shift throughout their lives. This may happen right before their menstrual period, when it is called *premenstrual syndrome*, or PMS. PMS is a pattern of disturbing physical, emotional, and behavioral symptoms that occur 1 to 2 weeks before the menstrual period and end when the period begins. Symptoms include anger, anxiety, depression, irritability, poor concentration, bloating, breast tenderness, fatigue, and muscle aches. A more severe form of PMS, called *premenstrual dysphoric disorder* (PMDD), has irritability as its main symptom.

PMDD has recently been linked to a set of genes on our chromosomes. This is big news in women's mental health because it shows that women who have PMDD have a basic difference in the way their cells respond to reproductive hormones. It's evidence that PMDD is not just a problem of unpredictable emotions and behavior that the woman should be able to control on her own, voluntarily. Until now, there has not been a lot of scientific evidence linking reproductive hormones and mood disorders; many providers accepted patients' accounts as valid anecdotal evidence for which there has been limited direct treatment. The evidence of a genetic link to PMDD also offers the potential for future treatment options in this and other reproductive hormone–related mood disorders.

Women may also experience depression during pregnancy or after childbirth, when it's known as *postpartum depression*. This depression is more than just the "baby blues." It is related to a rapid shift in reproductive hormones that a woman is experiencing. Symptoms of postpartum depression may be mild, with bouts of sadness and tearfulness, or deep and extreme. Untreated postpartum depression affects the health of the woman, infant, and rest of the family.

Episodes of depression are found in some women going through *menopause*, when the body naturally slows its reproductive hormone cycles and a woman stops having menstrual periods. When the ovaries start to decline in function, they make less estrogen (or *estradiol*). This drop in hormones may trigger depression in some vulnerable women. Symptoms can include fatigue, trouble sleeping, difficulty concentrating and remembering small details, hot flashes, night sweats, and mood shifts.

Depression at this time is called *perimenopausal, menopausal,* or *postmenopausal* depression. Menopause begins, on average, at age 47 and lasts 4 to 8 years. Perimenopause begins 3 to 5 years before menopause, when estrogen levels begin to slowly drop. Postmenopause occurs when a woman is in her 50s, when her monthly periods finally stop. Some women experience depression during these times. Episodes of depression can be less frequent and may sometimes disappear once a woman passes through menopause.

To find a potential association between hormone levels and your depression, use the Mood Chart (table 2.4) to track your moods. Make sure that you include the days of your menstrual cycle and other important events, such as the birth of a child, in the notes section on the chart. Then share the completed chart with your doctor.

Depression in a woman who is a wife or significant other, a mother, or pregnant can affect the entire family. Children growing up in a household where the mother has depression or bipolar disorder may experience a variety of emotional problems themselves. A spouse or significant other can also feel the effects.

The relationship between mood and hormones is not well understood, but research is ongoing. A valuable resource where you can learn more about current thinking and research on psychiatric issues throughout a woman's reproductive life is the website Women's Mental Health Across the Life Cycle, www.womensmentalhealth.org, operated by the Center for Women's Mental Health at the Massachusetts General Hospital, Boston. There you will find a library of information, a blog, and a newsletter of up-to-date topics on depression and PMS, perinatal and postpartum depression, fertility and mental health, and menopausal symptoms.

Depression in Men

Typically, adult men who have depression don't show the same degree of sadness, tearfulness, or hopelessness that is more common in women. Some men have irritability and agitation, rather than sadness, as their major symptom of a mood disorder. You may feel cranky and irritable instead of sad or tearful when depressed. Irritability can lead to angry outbursts or frustration toward others over minor matters. Sometimes, you just can't stand to be near other people. Some men may try to numb their pain with risky behaviors such as gambling, drinking, substance abuse, or engaging in excessive sexual behavior. Others work too much as a sign of depression, but they may not be doing a very good job.

Men may have more difficulty recognizing signs of depression in themselves and deciding when it is time to seek professional help. This may be because of social customs, social pressure, and cultural differences. In most societies, it is harder for men to admit to having emotional problems for fear of appearing weak, not macho, and in need of help. Men are often brought up to withhold their feelings. They often fear that friends, co-workers, supervisors, or teammates will find out and judge them poorly. This social stigma is misguided and unfortunate, and it adds to prolonged suffering.

Traditionally, researchers in psychiatry report that women experience symptoms of depression twice as often as men. Some wonder whether we are identifying all the instances of depression in men, because they may have a unique set of symptoms. In 2013 University of Michigan researchers looked at whether men and women experience depression in equal numbers. They gathered information using a self-reported questionnaire of English-speaking adults in the United States. The researchers found that symptoms such as anger, aggression, alcohol and substance use, irritability, and risk-taking behavior were more common in men than in women.

The researchers then combined these symptoms with fifteen "traditional" symptoms of depression in a new questionnaire rating scale. Men and women met the definition for depression in fairly equal numbers when measured with this combined rating scale. This suggests that our current methods of screening for depression might be missing symptoms common in some men, and that the data are under-reporting the instances of depression in men. More research is needed to better understand this.

Depression in Adolescents

Depression in a teenager is often different from that in an adult. Teenagers face extraordinary pressures from peers, school, family, or themselves, while also dealing with changing bodies, including in the body's balance of hormones, in a society that emphasizes body image, all of which can contribute to depression. Depression may be more common if there is a family history of a mood disorder, alcoholism, or suicide, or a history of early childhood trauma (physical or emotional).

Teenagers' exposure to social media 24/7 is a huge contributing factor in depression. Social media makes it hard to escape the need to be or to appear to be "perfect." As there is no firm line between their real and online worlds, adolescents can take on angst from others they have never met. Social media has led to technical and online bullying (for example, in Facebook, Instagram, or Snapchat entries), which can be malicious. Any form of bullying makes one feel like an outcast and a target, which can lead to depression and anxiety.

Irritability and agitation is a common feature of depression in a child or adolescent, sometimes the hallmark symptom. Daily habits, such as sleeping, eating, and social activities, may change without explanation. There may be a difference in school or work performance, a loss of friends or a new group of friends, or a change in activities once enjoyed. A teenager might be more withdrawn and secretive about what he does and where he goes and with whom. He may become argumentative and fight with parents or his siblings over minor things. Alcohol, illegal drugs, reckless driving, self-harm (like superficial cutting), and other reckless behavior are not uncommon as a way to cope with anxiety and depression.

A young woman may become tearful and highly sensitive, especially around the time of her menstrual period. Researchers are learning more about the biological link between reproductive hormones and depression. There's evidence that PMDD (premenstrual dysphoric syndrome) is related to genes and not just a problem of "unpredictable emotions" and behavior that she should be able to control on her own, voluntarily.

How does all this translate to depression in a teenager? You might see someone who has:

- stopped caring
- lost flavor for life, prior activities
- become hypersensitive to rejection and failure
- neglected appearance, dress, hair, hygiene
- changes in sleep and appetite, or weight
- become socially isolated, withdrawn
- irritability and is argumentative
- fatigue
- multiple vague physical aches and complaints
- shown evidence of self-harm (cutting) and reckless behavior
- changes in grades at school
- changes in social circle of friends—lost friends, new friends
- changes in types of activities involved in, including shift to drugs, alcohol

Which teenagers are at risk for depression? Depression is frequently seen in a person who experiences some of the following life problems, but having any of these is not a guarantee that the person will have depression:

- Issues that negatively affect self-esteem (obesity, severe acne, peer problems, bullying, academic problems)
- Experience as a victim of or witness to violence
- Learning disability or physical disability—anything that makes him feel different from peers
- Certain personality traits—low self-esteem, overly dependent, self-critical, or pessimistic
- Nontraditional gender roles in an unsupported environment (gay, lesbian youth)
- Family history of depression, bipolar disorder, or suicide
- Dysfunctional family life with conflict
- Living in a stressful neighborhood
- Stressful life event—parental divorce, illness, death, or military service; moving to a new home, neighborhood, or school

If you are a teenager and you notice any unusual changes in your typical emotions and behavior, it is important to talk to someone—a family member, school counselor, or clergy. Depression is treatable. Most often, treatment will be talk therapy with a counselor you choose and can trust. Sometimes medications are required as well.

You might have to make some changes in your life, such as staying away from toxic people who are not true friends and who steer you down an unhealthy path. You might also want to dial down your use of social media, or at least limit it to those close friends whom you know very well and who understand you and your illness, who won't be judgmental. Social media can be a pretty good way to stay in touch with your friends and what they're doing, but it's not as beneficial as face-to-face human contact. Remember that most people only put the "good stuff" on their social media profiles, so you get an exaggerated or biased view of their lives. That can make anybody feel bad. Nobody is partying and having a great time constantly. It's not fair to you to make comparisons with these unrealistic images. Avoid situations where these skewed images put extra pressure on you.

In addition, some teenagers may miss days of school or work or need to take a temporary leave of absence from school until they feel and function better, and that's okay. It's only a pause in the path of your life, and it is not as devastating as it might initially seem. As you feel better, you'll make up the time.

> The complications of *untreated* depression are that it can lead to alcohol and drug abuse, academic problems in school, family and social conflicts, involvement in the juvenile justice system, and suicide.

Depression in Older People

Depression is also very common in the elderly population. As people age, they often experience many of the familiar sources of depression. These include their own declining health problems and the loss of loved ones. Older people are at risk as they face

- loneliness,
- loss of friends, significant others, and family members,
- physical impairments that limit their lifestyle,
- medical problems,
- chronic pain, and
- loss of independence and purpose.

These problems do not always lead to depression, but when they do, it should be treated no matter the age.

In older individuals, the difference between depression and a natural grief response following the loss of a loved one can be difficult to sort out. Both include feelings of sadness and avoiding normal everyday activities, but with depression, the symptoms tend to be associated with constant negative thoughts, feelings of worthlessness, and low self-esteem. Depression can also be difficult to distinguish from dementia. Both are common in the older years and may be linked. The difference is that those who have depression are usually not disoriented like those who have dementia. People who have depression have difficulty concentrating, while those with dementia have problems with short-term memory. In depression, a person's writing, speaking, and motor skills are usually not affected as they are in dementia. If you have any questions about the diagnosis, your family doctor is the best resource to explore it further.

Sometimes there are obstacles to receiving treatment in older persons because they may regard depression as a weakness and are thus reluctant to seek professional help. Once the need for treatment is accepted, the choice of treatment may be difficult because older people are more likely to experience side effects of antidepressants. And these drugs may not interact well with their medications for other illnesses. For this reason, many older people quit or forget to take their medications due to side effects, underlying memory problems, or difficulty keeping track of complicated drug schedules. To avoid this problem, ECT (electroconvulsive therapy) is often recommended as a treatment in this age group.

Depression Accompanying Other Medical Problems

It may seem logical that people who have certain long-lasting medical problems may be prone to mood disorders. After all, they carry a large burden of stress in their medical illness, and stress stuck in overdrive can change the body and the brain. In some of these instances, people find themselves losing their lifestyle and purpose in life; their physical activities may be limited, and they might be in pain or in fear of losing their life. This can all affect mood in vulnerable individuals. Here are some examples of how medical problems can affect mood.

When your body makes too much thyroid hormone, mania can be triggered, while too little thyroid can lead to depression. Lack of vitamin B12 in the diet can lead to depression; this is common in the elderly. And up to 50 percent of those who have heart disease or certain types of cancer, such as breast cancer, will also face depression.

Other medical problems are associated with mood disorders:

- multiple sclerosis
- Parkinson disease
- Alzheimer disease
- Huntington disease
- stroke
- certain immune system diseases, such as lupus
- mononucleosis
- HIV

As if that isn't enough, some of the medications used to treat physical medical problems may lead to depression. The list includes some antimicrobials and antibiotics; heart and blood pressure drugs such as beta blockers (propranolol, metoprolol, or atenolol); calcium channel blockers (verapamil, nifedipine); digoxin; and methyldopa. Add to this list hormones like anabolic steroids, estrogens (Premarin), prednisone, and birth control pills. Then there are some miscellaneous drugs like clonazepam (Klonopin); cimetidine and ranitidine (Zantac); and narcotic pain medications. Withdrawal from cocaine or amphetamines may also cause depression.

The good news is that, similar to depression from all causes, depression related to long-term medical problems is treatable. The key is to recognize that it is happening and to seek professional mental health treatment early on. Some heart centers and oncology departments have mental health professionals on their team, ready to receive referrals from the treating physicians.

SYMPTOMS OF DEPRESSION

Depression affects your thoughts, feelings, and behaviors, which can interfere with the quality of your life. The most common symptoms include a
deep feeling of sadness; loss of interest and pleasure in your usual activities;
changes in appetite, weight, and sleep; loss of energy; fatigue; irritability;
feelings of worthlessness, hopelessness, and guilt; difficulty thinking, concentrating, and making decisions; and thoughts of suicide.

Table 2.2 provides examples of common thoughts, feelings, and behaviors related to depression. Check off those you can relate to and share this
information with your treatment team.

SYMPTOMS OF ELEVATED MOOD

The extremely elevated mood of bipolar disorder also affects your thoughts,
feelings, and behaviors, which can interfere with the quality of your life.
Table 2.3 provides examples of common thoughts, feelings, and behaviors
related to elevated mood. Put a checkmark next to those you can relate to
and share this information with your treatment team.

MOOD CHART

Use table 2.4 to record your mood every day, then share it with your provider. It's quick and easy to do. Check the box that best estimates your mood
for that day, such as a depressed or elevated mood that is severe, moderate,
or mild in intensity. Doing this will help you track fluctuations or identify
a pattern in your moods. Use the Notes column to record anything that
might have affected your mood—stressful events, medication changes, or
(in women) your menstrual period.

DEPRESSION AND ANXIETY

Approximately half of those who suffer from depression also suffer from
anxiety at the same time. This adds a great burden to the weight of feeling
depressed. Anxiety is a feeling of excessive apprehension, nervousness, and
worry about future events or activities. The depth of the anxiety or worry,
length of time it lasts, and how often it occurs is out of proportion to the

TABLE 2.2. **Symptoms of Depression**

NEGATIVE THOUGHTS

☐ I deserve this.

☐ I am being punished.

☐ It's all my fault.

☐ I can't make decisions.

☐ I can't remember anything.

☐ Nothing good will ever happen.

☐ Things will never get better.

☐ I never do anything right.

☐ I am not as good as everyone else.

☐ Nobody will ever care about me.

☐ I am worthless.

☐ People are against me.

☐ I should do/be _____.

☐ I have wasted my (life, education, opportunities).

☐ There is no hope for me.

☐ I think about dying or suicide a lot.

FEELINGS

☐ I feel sad for no reason.

☐ I don't feel good even if good things happen.

☐ I feel worthless.

☐ I feel bad, inferior to other people.

☐ I feel guilty about everything.

☐ I feel easily annoyed or irritable.

☐ I fear that something terrible will happen.

☐ I feel tired all the time.

☐ I am not interested in anything.

☐ I am not interested in sex.

BEHAVIORS

☐ I cry a lot for no reason.

☐ I sleep too much.

☐ I sleep too little.

☐ I eat too much.

☐ I eat very little.

☐ I drink too much alcohol.

☐ I recently gained a lot of weight.

☐ I recently lost a lot of weight without trying.

☐ I stay in bed or on the couch all day.

☐ Sometimes I don't take a shower, wash my hair, or shave.

☐ I have trouble starting or finishing projects.

☐ I avoid people and isolate myself.

☐ I do not return telephone calls.

☐ I have stopped my previous activities, hobbies.

☐ I stopped exercising.

☐ I argue and fight with people for no good reason.

☐ I am fidgety and restless.

☐ I move or speak slowly.

☐ I have trouble concentrating.

☐ I have difficulty reading the newspaper or following shows on TV.

☐ I can't keep track of my thoughts well enough to have a conversation.

☐ My house is more disorganized than usual.

☐ I forget to pay bills.

☐ I forget or don't do laundry or other household duties.

☐ I call in sick to work or school a lot.

TABLE 2.3. Symptoms of Elevated Mood

ELEVATED THOUGHTS

☐ I have special abilities.

☐ I have a lot of good ideas.

☐ My thoughts are really great.

☐ Many people are interested in me and my ideas.

☐ Many people are against me.

☐ I get very focused on a project or cause.

☐ My thoughts jump around quickly from one topic to another.

☐ Other people say they can't follow what I'm saying.

☐ The rest of the world is too slow.

☐ It takes others a really long time to do things.

FEELINGS

☐ I feel good even when bad things happen.

☐ I feel happy without reason.

☐ I am very self-confident.

☐ I have lots of energy even when I get less sleep than usual.

☐ I feel optimistic about everything.

☐ I feel great, on top of the world.

☐ I feel that everything will go my way.

☐ I feel that nothing bad can happen to me.

☐ I am easily annoyed or irritable.

☐ I am very impatient.

☐ I feel more interested in sex than usual.

BEHAVIORS

☐ I sleep less than usual and don't feel tired.

☐ I laugh a lot or for no reason.

☐ I am more talkative than usual.

☐ I am fidgety and restless, and I pace a lot.

☐ I have trouble concentrating.

☐ I am easily distracted.

☐ I start lots of new projects and activities.

☐ I have increased my activities, work, hobbies.

☐ I don't finish projects before starting new ones.

☐ I am much more sociable than usual.

☐ I make more phone calls than usual.

☐ I spend lots of money, go on shopping sprees.

☐ I make impulsive decisions.

☐ I tip excessively, gamble.

☐ I take more risks than usual.

☐ I do more risky or dangerous activities.

☐ I start arguments or fights for no reason.

☐ I drive fast.

☐ I increase my use of alcohol or drugs.

☐ I dress more flashy than usual.

☐ My handwriting is larger and messier.

TABLE 2.4. Mood Chart

Month: _____

DAY	DEPRESSED			NEUTRAL	ELEVATED MOOD			NOTES
	severe	moderate	mild	neutral	mild	moderate	severe	
1								
2								
3								
4								
5								
6								
7								
8								
9								
10								
11								
12								
13								
14								
15								
16								
17								
18								
19								
20								
21								
22								
23								
24								
25								
26								
27								
28								
29								
30								
31								

actual feared event and causes distress. The fear feels very real and scary at the time. The worry of anxiety is difficult to control and is often accompanied by other psychological or vague physical symptoms such as feeling restless or shaky, with difficulty concentrating, irritability, and disturbed sleep. You may feel nervous, jittery, worried, and sweaty, with your heart racing or skipping a beat, a headache, an upset stomach, and muscle aches.

Anxiety can be seen specifically as excessive worry about one's health; obsessive-compulsive disorder; social anxiety with fear of scrutiny by others and embarrassment when having to interact with others or perform; panic disorder, an episodic and abrupt onset of fear and physical symptoms; and anxiety associated with post-traumatic disorder.

It is thought that those who have generalized anxiety overestimate the level of danger in their surrounding environment, struggle with uncertainty in their lives, and underestimate their own capacity to cope. CBT, or cognitive behavioral therapy, can help a person restructure their thoughts to understand that their worry is not productive and can teach them relaxation skills.

People experiencing severe anxiety symptoms often go to the Emergency Department for fear that something physical is wrong. The good news is that many treatments for mood disorders, including those mentioned in this book, are also effective for treating anxiety. These treatments may include medications, talk therapy, mindfulness meditation, or a combination. CBT can help a person balance her fears and sense of danger in the world, deal with uncertainty, and learn effective coping skills. Lifestyle modifications, such as healthy sleep hygiene; avoidance of caffeine, tobacco, and alcohol; and deep breathing and relaxation exercises are also helpful.

THE STIGMA OF MOOD DISORDERS

Mood disorders such as depression and bipolar disorder still carry a stigma, even in the year 2018. A stigma arises when some misinformed people judge you because of your illness and then unfairly label you with a negative stereotype or image. This results in your being avoided, rejected, or shunned by others. Stigma can also be a barrier to your seeking professional help for your mental illness, if you fear that others may find out and judge you with a critical eye.

Some people may believe that it is socially unacceptable to have a mood disorder. They may try to make you feel ashamed or disgraced because of your illness. Others may believe you are incompetent, potentially dangerous, weak in character, or undesirable just because of your illness. They will be judgmental and critical of you. *But they are mistaken. Their beliefs are absolutely not true.*

There is nothing unacceptable about having a biologically based condition such as depression or bipolar disorder (or diabetes or heart disease, for that matter). Unfortunately, many people are not informed about mood disorders as an illness, and they believe in the stigma, the unfair criticism or judgment. They may try to force their inaccurate beliefs and attitudes on you. Ill-informed beliefs and judgments may come from your friends, family, or strangers who just don't know any better. These judgments may also come from the media, such as television or social media sites, which tend to sensationalize the news and perpetuate misconceptions. Remember that their misinformation is driving this behavior—it is not a reflection of you or the reality of mood disorders.

Some people you know may believe certain myths circulating around about mood disorders. These are often based on fear and lack of education about depression or bipolar disorder. Here are some examples:

- Mood disorders are contagious—another person can "catch it."
- People who have depression or bipolar disorder are violent or dangerous.
- Depression isn't a real illness. It just means you're weak or crazy.
- Depression is only a woman's illness. Men don't get it.
- You're doomed to get it because your parents had it.
- You can snap out of it if you want to.
- Antidepressant treatment alone is all you need.
- Antidepressants will change your personality.
- You will have to be on antidepressants forever.
- Talking about it will make things worse.

There is nothing true about these myths. The problem is that if believed, these myths can cause a person to feel more alone, troubled, and outcast. So it's important to question any statements like these that you might hear.

Having an illness with a stigma attached is an additional burden for you to carry on top of the depression symptoms you already feel. Having to deal with others' inaccurate reactions to and criticism of your illness can magnify the suffering you experience. You may feel you are constantly choosing whether to feel hurt and deal with that, or correct their misinformation, if you feel you have the mental energy to do so. When others attach a stigma to your illness, it can put a strain on your relationship with them at home, at work, or in social situations. Often, you need to step back and understand that you may never be able to turn around the other person's thinking no matter how hard you try. Consider what you know about the person—the source of their distorted beliefs—and try to ignore the comments of those whose opinion you cannot change.

FATIGUE AND DEPRESSION

Fatigue is a common symptom that affects people in both the general community and medical care settings, including psychiatry. It is considered to be a core symptom in mood disorders, affecting more than 75 percent of patients with major depression. Fatigue can significantly impair your ability to function and carry out your daily tasks. It may make it more difficult to get out of bed, get dressed, care for yourself or your family, prepare meals, or get out of the house to do errands or go to work. You may feel fatigue even when you think you are getting enough sleep, which can be quite frustrating.

What exactly is fatigue? There is no single definition. It is different from just feeling sleepy or tired. Fatigue can be thought of as a combination of symptoms, with three main dimensions: physical, mental, and emotional. You may have several of these together. The multiple components of fatigue have been described in this way:

Physical
- loss of energy
- heavy limbs
- persistent tiredness even without physical exertion
- exhaustion
- reduced activity tolerance
- decreased physical endurance, stamina
- increased effort to accomplish physical tasks
- generalized weakness
- slowness or sluggishness

Mental and cognitive
- mental dulling
- word-finding and recall problems
- problems focusing and sustaining attention
- difficulty concentrating
- decreased mental endurance
- slowed thinking

Emotional and psychological
- lack of motivation
- apathy, decreased interest
- weariness
- irritability
- boredom
- low mood

The various dimensions of fatigue are included in the *DSM-5* definition of depression, for example, physical fatigue (loss of energy), mental fatigue (difficulty concentrating), and emotional fatigue (loss of interest and pleasure, called *anhedonia*).

Depression-related fatigue has various possible causes, which may be difficult to sort out. But it is important to identify which one applies to you, if possible, so that you and your provider can address and treat the problem of fatigue effectively.

First, fatigue may be a *primary symptom* of your depression, along with other feelings of low mood, sadness, or loss of interest. Often the fatigue improves along with the treatment for depression. But fatigue can also be a *residual symptom* of depression, persisting after treatment in about 23 to 38 percent of people who are otherwise in remission. This means that, in some people, fatigue persists even after most other depression symptoms have improved or gone away following treatment with antidepressant medication. Residual fatigue can be difficult to resolve, but therapeutic options are available—speak with your psychiatrist if you are having persistent fatigue.

Next, fatigue can be a *side effect* of antidepressant medications, particularly some SSRIs (selective serotonin reuptake inhibitors). Sometimes this requires a change in medication to a different drug with fewer side effects, one that you tolerate better. Discuss medication changes with your treating psychiatrist. Remember to be specific about your side effect symptoms and how they affect the quality of your life.

Fatigue can also be related to *insomnia* and *poor sleep patterns*, which often occur along with depression. If this is a cause of your fatigue, CBT-I and adhering to good sleep hygiene practices will benefit you. Finally, fatigue may be related to *other medical problems* you may have. These problems may include diabetes; low thyroid condition; kidney, liver, lung, or heart disease; or others. These conditions do not necessarily cause the fatigue; there is just a potential association. In these cases, work with your treating physician to optimize your other medical conditions as much as possible.

What Helps with Fatigue?

Begin by investigating the conditions that may be contributing to your fatigue and work with your treatment team to modify what you can. You may need to avoid those antidepressant medications that are likely to worsen sleepiness and fatigue, choose antidepressant medications more likely to help resolve the symptoms, and consider using an additional medication that targets fatigue. Discuss these options with your psychiatrist.

Next, stick to the basics of mental health covered in the first chapter of this book. Remember to have regular nutritious meals, follow a regular sleeping and waking pattern (with a goal of getting 8 hours of sleep per night), take your medications as prescribed, avoid alcohol and illegal substances, maintain a daily routine and schedule, and keep up with social contacts. Then, even though it sounds difficult, get out and exercise a little every day, at a moderate level, based on your current ability. Yes, even when fatigued. You will be surprised how much exercise will improve your energy level.

Common Obstacles in Depression

With depression, feeling "good" is alien and may feel uncomfortable at first.
You are not used to it and may feel anxious. The brain sees it as different and
"not right," so the tendency is to go back. Don't. You have to push yourself.
—M. JACOBO

Depression commonly brings with it many obstacles, and they often seem so real at the moment that we often don't recognize them as barriers along our path. We come to accept them and are surprised to find they repeatedly trip us up. For example, obstacles to your healing from a mood disorder include feeling consumed by depression, having a fear of recovery, and ruminating. While not helpful to you or your recovery from depression, these ways of thinking are common. The first step is to recognize that your attention has drifted in this negative direction. Then you can take measures to lessen the effects of these obstacles on you.

FEELING DEFINED BY DEPRESSION

Depression is a biological illness, a set of symptoms. It does not *define* you. Depression is not what makes you "you," what makes you who you are. You are more than your depression, more than a set of symptoms. You have personality, character traits (such as kindness or a sense of humor), skills, abilities, and accomplishments that are unique to you. Perhaps you're capable or skilled in writing, sports, computers, or gardening. Maybe you're a good listener, friend, sister, or co-worker. Right about now, some of you are denying that you ever had any of these qualities in the first place.

With long-standing or repeated episodes of a mood disorder, the memory of "the person you are or have always been" can fade in your mind. Some of us may have difficulty remembering what we were like before depression hit us. We struggle to separate the symptoms of depression from our "regular self." It's easy to take on an "illness identity" of depression or have it overtake your life and then feel adrift in the symptoms. This might happen when a person has lost interest in life and forgets all else that he does or did, spending much of his time going to appointments, taking medications, dealing with his problems, and dropping everything else. Your life may become filled with feeling sad and miserable and working hard each day to manage the symptoms that have somehow overtaken your life. You may have little time, energy, or interest left for other things.

Some people who have depression or bipolar disorder feel, "This is not *me*—I don't feel familiar to myself." You might feel that you have lost your bearings. You then tend to forget who or what you were like before the illness, what you did with your time each day, what you were interested in or what made you smile. When someone reminds you, it doesn't seem to matter anymore. You might also forget about your preferences, interests, accomplishments, or the sense of yourself as a person. These are not permanently gone, just temporarily buried underneath an overwhelming array of illness symptoms you face each day.

The goal is to hold on to your usual sense of who you are and try not to get consumed by your depression symptoms. You might wonder how to do this.

To begin, recognize that depression is a biologically based illness of the mind and body. Yes, it does affect just about every aspect of your life, so you need to work hard to keep it in perspective *as an illness*. Having a mood disorder does change your life, but overall, it often ends up being in a more positive way for many people. How could I possibly say *that*? Well, for example, as your recovery approaches, you may end up viewing the world with a renewed set of goals and priorities, which can be good.

Another way to avoid becoming consumed by depression is to keep up with your baseline sense of yourself, your work, relationships, activities, and interests—the things that make you who you are, the thread of your life—despite having this illness. It's not easy to do; you may need the help of friends and family to remind you of who you are as a person and to help anchor you.

How do you do this? An easy exercise to help, called "Defining Your Baseline," is described in chapter 4. It helps you identify your strengths and weaknesses, personal preferences, beliefs, values, competencies, sense of purpose, and what nourishes and energizes you. It's a way to help you connect to your inner sense of yourself, to your baseline person. This is important to draw on as an aid in your recovery.

FEAR OF GETTING BETTER

Sometimes with a long-standing illness like depression or bipolar disorder, the idea of feeling better, or "good," may seem strange and uncomfortable at first. For this reason, some of us have an underlying fear of getting better, a fear of recovery. How can this be? Isn't that the ultimate goal, to feel better?

Fears are feelings surrounded by unhelpful thoughts; they are not *facts*. Fears may be based on faulty information or logic. Holding on to a fear can get in the way of making progress. You can learn to manage your "fear of getting better" just as you can learn to manage any other feelings in your life. One way is to try the "Mood and Thought Monitoring Exercise" in chapter 8.

When you are immersed in a mood disorder for a long time, the illness causes you to have a changed view of yourself and to adopt certain depressive behaviors that then become familiar to you. As you get used to experiencing a mood disorder, these depressed thoughts and actions become your new sense of "normal." Going back to feeling "good" then becomes strange and may cause you to feel uncomfortable at first. Since you are not used to it, you may feel anxious or irritable. The depressed brain sees feeling good as different and "not right," so the tendency is to go back to the thoughts, feelings, and behaviors of depression, irritability, or anxiety. Feeling depressed may feel safer and more comfortable than risking the new territory of wellness, which has a different (healthier) set of feelings, thoughts, and behaviors.

Recovery from a mood disorder doesn't just happen all at once, and it is not something to be feared. It has been defined by the Substance Abuse and Mental Health Services Administration (SAMHSA) as "a process of change through which individuals improve their health and wellness, live a self-directed life, and strive to reach their full potential." This means that recovery is an ongoing process in which you have a say in defining what your own improvement will look like and be. That is good.

> Think about recovery as an ongoing process of gaining control over your life after receiving a psychiatric diagnosis (and all the losses associated with that diagnosis, such as the loss of friendships or financial savings).

Recovery also means leaving behind the familiar illness and life as you know it *now*, venturing into the world of wellness that is probably uncertain and unfamiliar to you. That can be scary. You might feel anxious, irritable, and want to retreat back to your old depressed self. You don't know what to expect, especially if you've had trouble remembering what you were like before the depression began. So some people may feel more comfortable keeping things as they are, staying in the familiar depression. I urge you not to do this.

Some fear that when depression symptoms improve or go away, they will be at a loss in the way they think and act and view the world, believing that they won't know how to course through life in any different way. You will, though, because along the way you will have learned to replace the depressive symptoms and thoughts with a more positive view of yourself and the world, and that can help you approach life more confidently.

It takes a lot of work to get better. There is major effort required, and energy you may feel you won't always have. So you have to push yourself—push yourself beyond this, and eventually you will adjust to the idea of feeling better. After all, this is your ultimate goal. I urge you not to give up on yourself.

How to Address Your Fears

Here are some basic steps to help you better recognize your fears and address them. Write your answers down on a piece of paper and think about it for a little while.

1. Identify your specific fear.
2. Think about how it makes you feel (afraid, anxious, vulnerable, etc.).
3. What are the benefits of staying in your old comfort zone (not addressing the fear)?
4. What are the costs of not addressing your fear?
5. What are the benefits of addressing your fear?
6. What are the risks of doing this? What do you have to lose?
7. Identify a few small steps to address your fear.
8. Identify the support people you need to help you face your fear.
9. What resources do you need?
10. Begin to do a few of the small steps you just identified.

RUMINATION

Rumination is a state of having deep and repeated thoughts about something, such as thinking repeatedly about unpleasant experiences. Your attention is focused on the sources of your distress, not the solutions. It is a time when you may dwell on negative thoughts about past failures, with a focus on feeling inadequate or worthless. Sound familiar?

The dangers of rumination are that it can lead to experiencing increased anxiety and depression. It can also impair your ability to think through a situation clearly and interfere with problem solving. Ruminating is not productive.

How do you manage rumination? The first step is to recognize that it is happening, that your thoughts are not productive and that you feel like you're spinning your wheels, stuck in the mud. Then, try to interfere with the "rumination process" going on in your brain. How do you do this? You could try to distract yourself with activities, for example, a hobby or listening to music. More useful is to think of those challenging times when things turned out fine for you. Write them down so you have real-life examples available to remind yourself of your successes. Take steps to create more of these positive events in your life.

The next thing you want to do is identify and list the various *problems* that confront you at this moment. Problems can become intrusive thoughts that disturb you. This is rumination. Under each problem on your list, write down how you plan to address the problem: what steps you will take, what resources you need, whose assistance you must obtain. In planning your solutions, take small steps that are concrete, realistic, and measurable. Don't try to do something all at once. Once you have your list made, step back and take a look at it to see if there are any common themes among the problems you have to deal with. That may enable you to consolidate your efforts.

Then slowly begin to address your problems with the solutions you have outlined. Add to this list as new problems arise. If or when you find your thoughts drift to rumination, which you now understand is not productive, take steps instead to act on one of the problem-solving steps you have identified.

Defining Your Baseline

Practice consciously endorsing yourself.
—M. JACOBO

Your baseline is the way you feel when you're healthy and not depressed, manic, or anxious—it's the sense of who you are as a person. It reflects things like your interests, preferences, opinions, and accomplishments. Often depression can swallow you up, and you lose track of your baseline self. It feels like there is nothing *but* depression in life. Your time becomes filled with feeling sad and miserable, struggling each day to manage your symptoms. You may have little time or energy left for anything else. If you have long-standing or repeated episodes of a mood disorder, the memory of the person you are or have always been tends to fade in your disrupted mind. You're apt to forget what or who you were like as a person before the illness, what you did with your time each day, what you were interested in or what made you smile. Like me, you may struggle to sort out the symptoms of depression from "just me, my regular self."

In managing depression, you have to understand the difference between your symptoms and your true self. Having your baseline healthy self to draw on is an important aid during your recovery. This will help you envision what you are working toward. *You* are not your depression.

How do you do this, *stay connected to your baseline*? One way is with the following exercise. You can do this on paper or on a smartphone, tablet, or other electronic device of your choice. It's helpful if you have it in a handy place you can refer to occasionally.

Step 1. Create a list of your strengths and weaknesses, personal preferences, beliefs, values, skills, and competencies (tables 4.1 and 4.2).

Be realistic when you assess your strengths and weaknesses. Include your personal preferences, your likes and dislikes, needs, wants, skills, values, beliefs, opinions, sense of purpose, what nourishes you, energizes you, gives you pleasure and enjoyment or a sense of perspective and calm. Identify what makes life rich and full for you.

TABLE 4.1. **Strengths and Weaknesses Exercise**

This exercise is one of several steps to help you connect with your sense of self. In each column below, list your personal strengths and weaknesses. Be honest with yourself. Get feedback from others who know you well if you have difficulty doing this exercise.

MY STRENGTHS	MY WEAKNESSES

This exercise may be hard to do when you are depressed. You may feel as though you're describing another person. If you have difficulty with this, get feedback from others who know you well. Ask your friends and family to remind you, honestly, of your strengths and unique personal qualities.

Find a way to stay connected to your inner sense of yourself, to your baseline person, and not get consumed by your symptoms.

Once you identify these qualities, you will have a clearer idea of what you are about, which will help reconnect you to your healthy baseline self. Identifying your preferences and beliefs will help you *be* yourself. Use the worksheets in this chapter to guide you through this exercise.

Perhaps this example will help you get started. When I had trouble writing my own personal statement, my therapist used it as an illustration. In a scene from the movie *Bull Durham*, the baseball character played by the actor Kevin Costner gives us a modified version of this exercise when he confidently states: "I believe in the soul, . . . the hanging curve ball, high fiber, good scotch . . . I believe there ought to be a constitutional amendment outlawing Astroturf and the designated hitter . . . I believe in . . . opening your presents Christmas morning rather than Christmas Eve." He continues on to further list his preferences and opinions. Now we have a deeper idea of who the character is, what he values. Using that as an example, and with input from my friends, I made a list of my own preferences, personal qualities, and values, which we then discussed in session. That list eventually grew and became my responses to the Personal Preferences Exercise in table 4.2.

Step 2. Try to *do the things you like*, or used to like, to do.

Consciously choose more of your preferences that are "positive" and fewer of those that are "negative." Work to further develop your strengths and skills.

Step 3. Put together a brief statement about yourself, based on your strengths, beliefs, and preferences (box 4.1).

This is what you would say to yourself about yourself, your personal narrative. It is not for anyone else to hear right now. Describe who you are, your strengths, and your preferences. "I am a person who _____" is a good place to start.

Sit with it, get used to it, and practice saying it to yourself. Have that statement in your head so that you will have access to it when you need it. Then, when depression comes roaring in, you will have this reminder of who you are, a reminder that you are not defined by your depression. Eventually your personal narrative will feel comfortable.

Having self-confidence and opinions, having a sense of who you are, and having easy access to it also helps with your relationships.

Sample of a brief personal statement:

> I am a (man, woman) who is intelligent, considerate, and kind, with a subtle sense of humor, respected in my job, caring toward my parents, good at fixing bicycles, who values honesty, integrity, and friendship, and likes baseball, pasta, *Trivial Pursuit*, reading to my daughter, and mystery novels.

Now create your own.

My Personal Statement

I am a person who _____

_____

_____

_____

_____

_____

_____

_____

BOX 4.1. About Me

Sometimes I like myself because of my _____

_____

I have nice _____

I am good at _____

My best qualities are _____

My friends say that I _____

People say I have attractive _____

I feel good about myself when I _____

I really value _____

I believe in _____

I admire _____

_____ loves me.

_____ makes me feel good about myself.

I enjoy _____

_____ makes me feel calm and relaxed.

I look good in _____

I am content or happy when _____

My favorite place to go is _____

My favorite activity is _____

My favorite music is _____

My favorite movie is _____

My favorite book is _____

Add your own: _____

_____

_____

TABLE 4.2. Personal Preferences Exercise

WHAT I LIKE TO DO WITH MY TIME
Personal and family
Professional
Social and recreational
What would (or used to) give me pleasure?
What would (or used to) give me contentment?
What would (or used to) give me a sense of mastery and competence?

WHAT I WANT IN LIFE
Personal
Professional
Social

WHAT I DO NOT WANT IN LIFE
Personal
Professional
Social

(continued)

TABLE 4.2. Personal Preferences Exercise		
MY PREFERENCES	**MY PREFERRED**	**MY LEAST PREFERRED**
Social		
People (friends, relatives, etc.)		
Personal characteristics in a friend		
How I like to be treated		
Name I prefer to be called		
People I admire		
People who inspire me		
Topics and causes I care about		
Professional		
What I want from work		
What interests me? What do I like to do?		
I gain satisfaction from		
What kind of environment, workplace, do I like?		
My ideal job would be		

MY PREFERENCES	MY PREFERRED	MY LEAST PREFERRED
Personal		
Activities (What gives me energy? What is fun, interesting, relaxing?)		
Relaxation		
Smells, fragrances		
Colors		
Flowers		
Food		
Beverages		
Restaurants		
Plants, trees		
Seasons		
Views, scenery		
Pets, animals		

(*continued*)

TABLE 4.2. Personal Preferences Exercise

MY PREFERENCES	MY PREFERRED	MY LEAST PREFERRED
Exercise		
Sports (participate)		
Sports (watch)		
Vacation		

Art		
Art, artists		
Museums		
Architecture		
Books, authors		
Magazines, newspapers		
Columnists, reporters		
Music—type, performers, composers		
Movies		
Actors		

MY PREFERENCES	MY PREFERRED	MY LEAST PREFERRED
Television		
Theater, plays		

Personal Style		
Clothing, jewelry, shoes		
Designers		
Shops		
What kind of home do I like?		
Location—where would I like to live?		
Weather, climate		
Style, architecture of home		
Interior style—furniture, color, texture		
Objects in home		
Car, truck, other vehicle		

5

Managing Your
Mood Disorder

We cannot direct the winds, but we can adjust our sails.
—THOMAS S. MONSON

FOLLOW YOUR TREATMENT PLAN

Treating your depression and bipolar disorder is ideally a collaborative effort between you and your doctors and often includes both medication and talk therapy, also called psychotherapy. Most people seek treatment to feel better and to function better. Treatment can also help you learn new skills, understand and manage your emotions, and deal with difficulties in your relationships.

Decisions made in partnership with your treatment providers is called *shared decision making*. It is the model of patient-centered care, a process in which the clinician and you as the patient work together to make decisions and to select diagnostic tests, treatments, and care plans based on clinical evidence while balancing the risks and benefits with your personal preferences and values. Your physician and therapist, who respect your goals and preferences, will use them to guide their recommendations and treatments.

Why should you get involved in these decisions? First, the more you understand your options, the better you will be able to follow through on recommendations. You have input. You feel respected. It also helps to build a trusting relationship with your clinician. Note that you must take some responsibility for speaking up to share your concerns, goals, and questions and to seek out information when offered. For more on this, I direct you to the AHRQ website (Agency for Healthcare Research and Quality) at www .ahrq.gov.

Most people with depression or bipolar disorder are treated in an outpatient (office) setting. Usually, a psychiatrist is the doctor who prescribes medication and works with you to create an overall treatment plan. In most cases, your PCP or family doctor makes a referral for you to see a psychiatrist or clinical psychologist. But in some cases, an internist or a family doctor prescribes your medication. Table 5.1 provides a helpful list of "who's who" in an outpatient depression treatment team.

If you don't have access to a primary care physician to make a referral, you can always contact your local mental health center or the patient referral telephone line in the Department of Psychiatry at your local community or university hospital. They can match you up with an available clinician suited to your symptoms.

TABLE 5.1. **Who's Who in an Outpatient Depression Treatment Team**	
Psychiatrists	Medical doctors who are specialty trained in psychiatry; licensed and board certified to treat mental illnesses such as depression, bipolar disorder, anxiety, and other conditions. They can evaluate individuals for a disorder and prescribe medications such as antidepressants.
Psychologists	Mental health clinical specialists who have obtained their master's degree or PhD in clinical psychology and who are trained and licensed to evaluate and treat using various kinds of talk therapy. Psychologists are sometimes referred to as therapists.
Social workers	Licensed clinical social workers (LICSW or LCSW) are trained to provide talk therapy to individuals or groups of people.
Nurse practitioners	Some nurse practitioners (NPs), those with advanced training who specialize in psychiatric disorders, may be licensed to prescribe antidepressants and other medications.
Psychiatric nurses	A nurse who specializes in psychiatry, in helping those who have mental health problems, may be part of your team on an inpatient unit and in some outpatient centers.

As mentioned in chapter 2, there continues to be a stigma about depression and other mental illnesses. Remember that this stigma is based on false information and don't let it affect your decision to seek professional help for your illness.

TALK THERAPY

Psychotherapy (talk therapy) is a cornerstone treatment for mood disorders. Alone or combined with medication, it has been effective in relieving and preventing further episodes of depression. Talk therapy is a type of guided therapeutic conversation that focuses on your psychological and emotional problems, distorted thinking, and troublesome behaviors. It can help you cope with your illness, understand yourself better, learn healthy ways to manage stress, make sound life decisions, and adjust to major life losses and transitions. Talk therapy can be done one to one or in a group setting.

The mental health professional who specializes in talk therapy is usually a *clinical psychologist* or *clinical social worker*, who will work with you to create a psychotherapy treatment plan. The success of psychotherapy depends on building a trusting relationship with a therapist who is a good fit for you. Psychotherapy takes time and effort to see results. It is not a passive treatment—you need to do a lot of hard work to gain from it. Sometimes you benefit from the work you do during appointments (individual or group therapy). Often the benefits come from work you do during the rest of the week, when you have the opportunity to apply to your daily life what you have learned in your sessions.

Treatment often involves making some change in the way you think or behave, and that may be uncomfortable. Changing to something unfamiliar can be both scary and hopeful. It is scary because you are doing something different and perhaps outside your comfort zone, and hopeful because the purpose is to feel better. Psychotherapy may also stir up unpleasant emotions. Dealing with these emotions is important to your recovery.

There are many different types of psychotherapy, each with a different name. The type you receive depends on your problems and your needs.

Cognitive behavioral therapy (CBT) is a form of talk therapy that has been extensively tested and shown to be very effective in treating depression and reducing the risk of relapse (return of symptoms). CBT addresses the connection between our thoughts, feelings, and behaviors. You learn to identify and change distorted thinking patterns, inaccurate beliefs, and unhelpful behaviors. You can read more on CBT in chapter 8.

Mindfulness-based CBT is a somewhat different approach that is also effective for some people. It has a focus of being in the moment, not dwelling on past or future events.

Dialectical behavior therapy (DBT), another type of psychotherapy, teaches concrete cognitive behavioral and mindfulness skills in four modules: (1) mindfulness, (2) interpersonal effectiveness, (3) emotion regulation, and (4) distress tolerance. It has been shown to be an effective additional therapy to antidepressant medication, resulting in improvement in depressive symptoms.

Medication therapy and psychotherapy alone are each effective in treating depression and reducing the risk of relapse and recurrence. In combination, they offer an even greater benefit against relapse. They are seen as therapies that complement each other. Psychotherapy offers a broader range of benefits than antidepressants do, such as improving your level of functioning, diminishing residual symptoms, targeting specific symptoms (such as guilt, hopelessness, and pessimism), teaching coping skills, improving interpersonal relationships, and targeting different brain sites. The effects of psychotherapy are longer lasting and sustained beyond the end of treatment.

MEDICATIONS

Depression is often treated with an antidepressant medication. Bipolar disorder may be treated with mood-stabilizing medications, such as lithium or others. A list of some typical drugs used to treat mood disorders can be found in the appendix at the back of this book. Each person is different and may require a different medication or a combination of medications. Research has shown that the most effective treatment is a combination of talk therapy and medication. Mild symptoms may respond well to either talk therapy or medication alone.

It may take 6 to 8 weeks after starting a medication for you to begin to see improvement and feel like yourself again. Sometimes, you have to try several different ones before finding the most effective medication or combination of medications for you. About one-third of people don't respond to the first medication they try, so it's important for you to keep working with your doctor to find the best plan for you.

It's essential to stay on the medication once your symptoms have started to improve. Stopping it too soon puts you at risk for recurrence (return) of your symptoms. This does not mean that you are dependent on the drug.

Unfortunately, research has shown that nonadherence (not sticking) with antidepressant medication is a common problem, with only half of patients continuing an adequate dose of therapy in the short term. Those patients are at risk for not getting better or for having their symptoms return. This is why it is important to continue to see your physician, preferably a psychiatric specialist, regularly until your symptoms clear.

For those who are uninsured or have demonstrated financial need, there are some patient assistance programs for obtaining medications. These programs provide prescription medications at little to no cost to you. One resource is Partnership for Prescription Assistance (www.pparx.org). Established in 2005, they offer a free service with access to 475 public and private programs, including 200 biopharmaceutical (drug) companies. Eligibility varies. Another organization is Prescription Hope. You may also contact some of the drug companies directly.

INPATIENT CARE

Sometimes the symptoms of your mood disorder worsen to the point where treatment in an inpatient hospital setting is needed. Inpatient care is a more intense form of treatment, where you receive daily individual and group therapy as well as medication management. Entering the hospital can be a scary experience the first time you are admitted, especially when you do not feel well and do not know what to expect. It can also be difficult if you do not feel the support of family or friends, who may not understand your illness or its treatment. Yet, an inpatient unit provides a safe environment during a rough time. This is especially important for those who have disorganized or suicidal thoughts. Most people treated in a hospital find it to be extremely helpful and even lifesaving.

On the inpatient unit, you work with a team of mental health professionals who review your current treatment plan and may suggest modifications. The inpatient team usually includes a senior psychiatrist, psychologist, nurse, social worker, and sometimes an occupational therapist. A teaching hospital will also have psychiatry residents, medical students, and sometimes nursing students. Your inpatient treatment plan is a collaborative plan between you and your team; you have the right to decide what feels appropriate and helpful for you, as long as it is safe. In some cases, treatments such as ECT (electroconvulsive therapy, also called shock therapy) may be recommended as part of your plan. You will also receive the support and input of other patients in group therapy sessions.

What if you are *afraid or reluctant to receive treatment?* A person may be uncomfortable or concerned about starting medication or psychotherapy treatment for both valid and faulty reasons. Sometimes these decisions are based on misinformation or anecdotal stories heard from others, in the news or on social media. These are not reliable sources of information on which to base your decision. Some of the reasons for treatment reluctance are:

- believing the need for treatment indicates you are a failure—*not true!*
- not wanting to feel more vulnerable and believing that talk therapy is intrusive, that your problems are "private"—*your therapist is trained to help you with this*
- feeling concerned about financial issues in paying for treatment—*there is financial assistance available for those who need it*
- being worried about privacy issues and fear of stigma if friends or co-workers find out—*okay, not everyone you know is educated about mental illness*
- believing that treatment is not effective, at least for you—*there are many types of treatment, and your providers will choose a plan to suit your needs*
- not being familiar or comfortable with mental health issues because of age or cultural background—*this requires education about mood disorders as a biological illness*
- having a fear of becoming dependent on medications—*not likely*
- dreading certain side effects you have heard rumors of—*anticipation is often worse than real life*
- feeling concerned that treatment such as talk therapy may raise up strong emotions that you fear having to deal with—*your therapist is trained to help you deal with this*

The best way to address these concerns is with solid information about the illness and proven treatment options from reliable sources. Then talk about your fears and worry with an experienced mental health clinician. You can go for a consultation without having to agree to treatment right away, and you can have a discussion with your provider in which you share information and treatment decisions. In most cases, the anxiety and reluctance will fade away.

WHAT TO DO WHEN YOU CAN'T AFFORD TREATMENT

Many countries offer comprehensive health care programs that include mental health services. Despite the foundations of the Affordable Care Act, more and more people in the United States find they are unable to afford professional mental health services. If this is true for you, what are your options? Here are a few:

- *In-training programs* at university teaching hospitals, where clinical care is provided by residents-in-training who are supervised by senior psychiatry staff members.
- *Sliding scale clinics* where the fee for mental health services is adjusted on a sliding scale for those who have documented financial need.
- *Pro bono (free)* care from some mental health professionals—this care depends on the individual provider, and eligibility varies.
- *School clinics*, where mental health care, usually short term, is provided by counselors in high schools and colleges, often for free or at a reduced rate.
- *Community services*, such as mental health clinics offered by state, federal, and local health departments for those in financial need (see a list of these at CDC.gov).
- *Referral to low-cost services* through the NAMI (National Alliance on Mental Illness) website (www.NAMI.org) or by calling 1-800-950-6264.
- *Listing of free mental health clinics* provided by SAMHSA (Substance Abuse and Mental Health Services Administration) at SAMHSA.gov.
- *Employment-based Employee Assistance Programs* (EAPs) provide mental health services to employees for free (for several sessions) or at a reduced rate—check with your employer.
- The *National Suicide Prevention Lifeline* at 1-800-273-8255 offers emergency assessment.

For those who live in rural areas, access to mental health professionals is often a problem. While Medicare has authorized Telehealth for certain medical visits, a virtual visit may not lend itself very well to the care of those who have a mood disorder or other psychiatric illness. Reimbursement varies, but it may be covered. There are licensure issues when care is provided across states. And there are significant privacy concerns. Most of all, a virtual visit does not allow for the patient-therapist relationship to develop. That bond is the key to successful therapeutic treatment, and without a private, safe place in which to communicate openly, the therapy is jeopardized. Telehealth may be useful as a tool to use in-between face-to-face appointments, or in remote geographic areas; research is ongoing.

You can learn to manage your illness in this and the next few chapters.

THE RELATIONSHIP WITH YOUR THERAPIST

The success of your treatment, particularly psychotherapy, depends on building a trusting relationship with a therapist who is a good fit for you. How do you find this therapist? That answer varies among individuals. One place to start is to ask your psychiatrist or primary care doctor for a recommendation. Depending on who is available in your geographic area, you may be referred to a clinical psychologist, licensed therapist, or licensed clinical social worker. Try to find one who specializes in treating patients with depression or bipolar disorder. If you live near a large teaching hospital, most academic psychiatry departments have a specialized Depression Unit that can refer you to a staff member. Get several names and then interview each one *face to face* to see if you feel comfortable speaking with this person. Not everyone will be a good match for you, so keep looking until you find someone you think will work.

Don't be afraid to ask questions of the people you interview: Inquire about their professional training and background. Make sure that the person you choose will coordinate your care with your other doctors (psychiatrist, family doctor, etc.). Find out if the therapist can schedule your appointments around your work hours. Ask about the method of payment and whether or not your health insurance company will pay for it. Ask if the person has particular experience with your cultural background and primary language. If you live in a remote area, check out whether the therapist can communicate with you by telephone or through a Skype session or other online options.

> In addition to taking medications and participating in psychotherapy, taking steps to manage your illness in your everyday life is essential. Helping yourself in this way offers the best chance of recovery and of staying well.

What Makes a Good Therapist?

There are many different therapists, each with a particular style, personality, and training. They may also practice different types of psychotherapy. Those differences do not prevent them from delivering good quality care.

You should expect that a good therapist

- listens and pays attention
- is empathetic and understanding
- is not judgmental or dismissive
- shows respect
- builds trust over time
- offers sound professional advice
- maintains boundaries
- does not impose his or her personal biases or viewpoints on you
- helps you to see your way through a problem and does not do it for you
- builds on your strengths
- offers you a regular appointment at the same time and day
- begins and ends appointments on time
- does not take telephone calls or allow other distractions during your appointment
- is available to you by page or telephone after hours for emergencies
- maintains your privacy and confidentiality

What Makes a Good Patient?

What do you need to do to get the most benefit from your therapy? Show by your actions that you are interested in and committed to talk therapy. Participating in therapy is a two-way street, and you have to do a lot of the work. You also need to keep up a good professional relationship with your therapist. Helping yourself in this way provides the best chance of recovery and of staying well.

These guidelines will help you be successful in therapy:

- Follow all treatments as prescribed. This includes taking medications and acting on other recommended therapies.
- Keep your appointments as scheduled. Do not skip appointments or cancel them at the last minute unless there is an emergency.
- Go to your appointments on time and stay for the entire session.
- Arrive sober. Do not show up to your appointment under the influence of alcohol or drugs.
- Be honest with your therapist.
- Make an effort.
- Do the "homework" assignments that your therapist asks you to do.
- Come prepared for each session with an idea of what you would like to discuss or work on with your therapist.

- Turn off your cellphone, tablet, and other electronic devices during your appointment.
- Listen.
- Pay attention to the conversation. Catch yourself if you begin to daydream off the subject.
- Take notes if you are having trouble concentrating or remembering what is being discussed.
- Show respect.
- Maintain boundaries. This is a professional relationship, not a casual friendship.
- Control your anger and outbursts during the session. If anger is a problem for you, your therapist will make addressing it part of your treatment plan.
- Learn to trust the therapist and understand that he or she has your best interest in mind.
- Avoid making phone calls to your therapist unless the situation is urgent.
- Call your therapist or go to the nearest Emergency Department if you are feeling unsafe or suicidal.

MANAGING DEPRESSION AND BIPOLAR DISORDER

Managing your depression or bipolar disorder effectively is critical to maintaining your emotional balance and stability. It can help you feel and function better. Research studies consistently show that people who participate actively in their care and work to manage their illness have a better chance of recovery and of staying well. Some people find that the symptoms of depression interfere with what they must do to manage their illness. For example, the symptoms of fatigue, poor appetite and sleep, and lack of interest can interfere with your ability to get the physical exercise necessary for a healthy life. This makes managing your illness a challenge, but it can be done. And it will make a difference.

What does it mean to *manage your illness*? It means that you learn about the illness and that you use certain methods, strategies, and skills each day to respond to the symptoms you have. These strategies are discussed in detail in this chapter. Developing the tools to deal with your illness will help you recover, prevent worsening, and avoid relapse (a return of symptoms).

Managing your depression effectively requires that you pay attention to your symptoms and monitor them, challenge negative thoughts, use problem-solving techniques, make adjustments, and avoid negative behaviors (see chapter 7). It means that you regulate your daily routine and make efforts to improve current relationships. Effective management also includes attending to self-care, following a healthy lifestyle and diet, getting physical exercise, and following the treatment plan you developed with your provider.

Self-management is best done in collaboration with your health care providers, who work with you and guide you along the way. You need to be partners in the process and participate in making decisions about treatment, interpreting and managing changes in your condition, coping with emotional reactions, implementing behavioral changes, and using medical and community resources wisely. Actively managing your illness may enable standard therapies to work better and may decrease the risk of relapse.

BOX 5.1. Managing Depression and Bipolar Disorder

Living with depression is a lot of hard work. For the best chance of success, you will need to take the following steps:

- Accept it as an illness.
- Follow your treatment plan.
- Understand the fluctuations (changes) in your symptoms and your symptom patterns.
- Define your baseline.
- Identify and monitor your triggers (chapter 7).
- Identify and monitor your early warning signs and symptoms (chapter 7).
- Develop an Action Plan to use when things get worse, when you or others notice your warning signs (chapter 7).
- Use relapse prevention strategies. Relapse prevention is a day-to-day approach to help you stay well (chapter 7).
- Learn and use effective coping skills (chapter 9).
- Maintain social connections. Avoid isolation.
- Maintain self-care.
- Stick to a daily routine and structure. Schedule your time.
- Do something every day, even when you don't feel like it.
- Build mastery (chapter 8).
- Develop a tolerance for feeling distress for a short time, during a moment of crisis (chapter 9).

Research has shown an improvement in depression symptoms when patients collaborate with their providers, are educated about the illness, share decision making about medications, and use cognitive behavioral strategies to promote self-management. These strategies include keeping track of depression symptoms, monitoring yourself for early warning signs, socializing, engaging in pleasant activities, and developing a written self-care plan for situations that could lead to a worsening or recurrence of depression. Another study showed the importance of these factors in helping people with mood disorders stick with taking their antidepressant medications, which contributes to better depression outcomes.

Managing your mood disorder involves the following steps (which are also listed in box 5.1).

Acceptance

Accept your depression or bipolar disorder as an illness, an illness that affects your body and your mind. It is not a weakness or a character flaw, or something that you have complete control over. It is an illness that can be treated and managed in a way that minimizes the effect of the illness on the quality of your life. Sometimes family or friends have a different opinion about your mood disorder or try to help by offering suggestions that are unfortunately misinformed. *Do not listen to these differing viewpoints.*

Follow Your Treatment Plan

The treatment plan developed by your providers, with your input and approval, is designed to help you. Take all medications as prescribed, and notify your doctor if you take any over-the-counter or nonprescription drugs. Keep taking your medications even after your symptoms have started to improve, and do not change the dose. Avoid alcohol and street drugs, which will only worsen your symptoms. It is also important to actively participate in your therapy sessions, do your prescribed homework exercises, and not skip appointments.

Understand Your Fluctuations (Ups and Downs)

Fluctuations are changes in your symptoms over time. You *will* have fluctuations up and down at different times during this illness. Use the Mood Chart (table 2.4) to identify them. From looking at this chart and working with your therapist, learn to understand the fluctuations in your symptoms and the patterns that you have. When you are experiencing an episode of depression, remembering that things will change for the better is hard. Try to remind yourself of this during those dark times. Aim to minimize the depth, intensity, and duration of your symptoms by working with your therapist and using the suggestions in this book.

Define Your Baseline

With depression or bipolar disorder, you may have trouble remembering anything but your current mood state. Find a way to stay connected to your sense of who you are, your inner sense of self. Remembering your baseline self, or healthier state of mind, will help you keep each episode in context, and you will feel more in control of your life. You are not your depression.

Having a clear image of your baseline healthy self to draw on during your recovery will help you know what you are working toward. You may need to ask people who know you well to help you. Ask your friends or family to remind you honestly of your strengths and unique personal qualities, then write them down. Review that list periodically. See chapter 4 for an exercise to help you do this.

Identify and Monitor Your Triggers

Triggers are events or circumstances that may cause you distress and lead to an increase in your symptoms. Being aware of what can worsen your symptoms is crucial to avoiding relapse (see page 106). You may not be able to change the trigger itself, but you can learn to modify how you respond to it so that you do not feel as much distress. Work with your therapist to identify, monitor, and modify your response to your triggers.

Identify and Monitor Your Early Warning Signs and Symptoms

Warning signs are distinct changes from your baseline that precede an episode of depression or mania (see page 107). Each person has a characteristic pattern of warning signs. These are changes in your thoughts, feelings, behaviors, routine, or self-care that are noticeable to you or others. Being aware of the changes that are warning signs for you will help you recognize the episode early. This will give you a chance to intervene and change the course of the depression or bipolar episode.

Symptoms that might be warning signs are those characteristic of depression or mania that last for two weeks or longer (see chapter 2). They may include changes in appetite, sleep, thinking, or concentration; loss of interest; sad, worthless, hopeless, or guilty feelings; negative or elevated thoughts or feelings; or behavior that is slowed down, irritable, restless, or overactive.

Develop an Action Plan

An intervention Action Plan for Relapse Prevention is a written self-care plan to help you deal with a worsening or a recurrence of depression. It outlines the steps you will take to manage, cope with, and distract from the intensity of a depressive or manic episode. In your plan, you also list the people you will ask to help you: health care providers, family, and friends. Work with your therapist to develop an intervention Action Plan to use when things get worse, when you or others notice your warning signs or a change in your emotional state. Create your Action Plan now and have it ready to use before you have any intense symptoms. See table 7.1 for a sample Action Plan for Relapse Prevention.

Use Relapse Prevention Strategies

Relapse prevention is a day-to-day approach to help you stay well. It is a way for you to identify, monitor, and respond early to changes in your symptoms. The approach also involves daily preventive steps to strengthen your emotional resources. For more information on relapse prevention, see chapter 7. A relapse prevention strategy includes five main steps that you and your treatment team will act on:

1. Identify in advance what your warning signs are.
2. Pay attention to your warning signs. Notice when changes from baseline begin to show.
3. Have an Action Plan prepared in advance and ready to use when your symptoms change.
4. Follow daily prevention steps to help you remain stable.
5. If you notice a change in your emotional health, follow your Action Plan. The plan will enable you to intervene early and modify or improve the course of the episode.

Use Coping Skills

Coping skills are the actions we take to lessen the effect of stressors and to get us through difficult times. These skills include problem solving, self-soothing, distraction, relaxation, humor, and managing the little things before they get too big. Learning and using effective coping skills are essential to managing your mood disorder. Coping skills are discussed in more detail in chapter 9.

Connect

Maintaining social connections is important to everyone's emotional health. It can be difficult to do on your own when depressed, so enlist the help of friends and family to stay in touch with you. Being with people you like has a positive effect on your mood. It gives you a sense of acceptance, increased self-esteem, a chance for friendship and fun, and access to people who can support you when needed. Avoid isolation and withdrawal because they will only worsen your depression. Some people find help in support groups with people who share the same illness and concerns.

Maintain Self-Care

Get up, take a shower, shave, wash your hair, and brush your teeth. Every day. Get dressed in clean, nice clothes and avoid wearing sweat pants all day long. Get a haircut or a manicure without feeling guilty. Doing so does not diminish the seriousness of your illness. These activities may sound simple, but they require a lot of energy and are challenging to do when depressed. They may also be the last things you are interested in doing. But taking good care of your body will help you feel better about yourself. Don't forget to give yourself credit for these accomplishments.

Stick to a Daily Routine and Structure

Having a daily routine and structure can help in many ways, such as helping you to avoid spending endless hours of empty alone time, which will only worsen your symptoms of depression (see page 33). It also gives you a purpose to your day, which will help improve your self-esteem. Schedule your time and try to follow that schedule, but don't be too rigid with yourself. Many people with depression struggle with their daily activities. Following a written schedule helps you to see and stick to everything you need to do, which feels good and is a daily accomplishment.

Do Something Every Day

With depression, your motivation to do anything seems to disappear, especially with how difficult everything seems to be during an episode. You may not feel like doing anything, but try anyway—at least *one* thing. Action precedes motivation. Do something every day, even when you don't feel like it. Interest in doing it will come later.

Build Mastery

Mastery involves doing something that is a bit difficult and that challenges you a little. This may be learning a new skill or hobby, or overcoming an obstacle. When you work on a mastery activity, you will feel more competent and effective, and you will gain a sense of achievement (see pages 34, 126, and 133). Give yourself credit for trying.

Develop Distress Tolerance

Distress tolerance strategies involve using skills to help you get through the crisis of a difficult moment. These skills include distracting yourself, soothing yourself, providing solace, and improving the moment itself (see pages 140–42). In a crisis you may sometimes feel a sense of urgency or a desire to act impulsively. This can interfere with your efforts to manage depression and remain stable. Working to develop your tolerance for distress over a short period can help you get through the rough moments.

ADDITIONAL TIPS FOR MANAGING YOUR MOOD DISORDER

Here are some additional pointers from the Joint Commission's 2013 educational program for those who have depression. The Joint Commission is an independent nonprofit organization that evaluates, accredits, and certifies nearly 21,000 health care organizations and programs in the United States to meet certain performance standards. Their program is called Speak Up: What You Should Know about Adult Depression (www.jointcommission .org/topics/speak_up_depression.aspx). Their goal is to help people become better informed about the common warning signs of depression, how to get the most out of your treatment, and how to speak up if a loved one needs professional care. The Speak Up program urges people to take an active role in their own health care. The educational material in the Speak Up brochures urges you to:

- **S**peak up if you have questions or concerns, and if you don't understand, ask again. It's your body, and you have a right to know.
- **P**ay attention to the care you are receiving. Make sure you're getting the right treatments and medications by the right health care professionals. Don't assume anything.
- **E**ducate yourself about your diagnosis, the medical tests you are undergoing, and your treatment plan.
- **A**sk a trusted family member or friend to be your advocate.
- **K**now what medications you take and why you take them.
- **U**se a hospital, mental health clinic, or other type of health care organization that has undergone a rigorous on-site evaluation against established state-of-the-art quality and safety standards, such as those provided by the Joint Commission.
- **P**articipate in all decisions about your treatment. You are the center of the health care team.

What Is the Goal?

Health is a state of complete physical, mental and social well-being,
and not merely the absence of disease or infirmity.
—WORLD HEALTH ORGANIZATION

When you find yourself in the midst of depression or bipolar disorder, what is it that you want? What do you expect to get from treatment? What is the goal? If you ask most people who have a mood disorder, they would say that topping the list of what they want is to feel better. But what is "better"? To most, it means that the symptoms of depression have gone away. Yet the absence of symptoms is not enough for you to feel *well*. Being well is not only freedom from the episodes of a mood disorder or depressive symptoms. It's an ongoing process that includes participating in the world around you, being in control of your life, having a sense of personal growth, and having relationships that matter. It means that you have a sense of competence and mastery in the things you do in your life and that you feel good about who you are.

WELLNESS AS THE GOAL

There is an interesting article on psychological well-being by Professor C. D. Ryff, from the University of Wisconsin–Madison, called "Psychological Well-Being Revisited: Advances in Science and Practice." In the past, psychologists thought of well-being as happiness, satisfaction with life, and a positive affect (similar to mood). Thinking about well-being more deeply, Ryff describes the essential features in this way:

- *Having a purpose in life*, feeling your life has meaning and direction. You might find this in your work or volunteer activities, as a student, parent, or in whatever role guides you. Our purpose is easy to forget when we're depressed, so we do have to work on it.

- *Living a life based on your own personal convictions*, beliefs, opinions, and principles. This means you are free to make decisions for yourself (called *autonomy*). For example, if you are an adult, do you feel controlled by another person, or respected for your thoughts, opinions, and decisions?
- *Making use of your personal talents and potential*, also called *personal growth*. This growth could occur in your work, school, volunteering, or family life.
- *Managing your life situations well*, also called mastering your environment. We all experience fluctuations, the ups and downs of daily life: the key is how we learn to deal with them.
- *Having positive relationships*, with deep ties to others. Your close personal connections could be with friends or family members—just as long as you have them. These relationships are very important to maintaining your mental health balance and definitely help with depression, a time when isolation can occur.
- *Accepting yourself*, which means having knowledge and acceptance of who you are as a person, including your own limitations. Nobody's perfect—we all have our own strengths and weaknesses, and we do better when we learn to accept and work with them.

Wow! You might now be thinking, *How in the world can I be well if I have to achieve all of these things? I've always been a loser—this won't happen to me!* I agree that these goals are difficult for anyone to achieve, let alone someone who has a mood disorder. Psychological well-being is not the kind of thing that happens overnight; it takes a lot of time and effort on your part. And you don't have to master them all at once.

STEPS TO WELLNESS

You might begin by trying to identify one or two areas in your life from this list that you want to work on. Your therapist can help you with this. Put those two areas into a clearly stated goal, like *I want to have my own opinions and control over the decisions in my life*. Having a goal set in this way helps you to achieve the kind of life you want. Think of your strengths, of past successes you have had in this area, and use these to boost your confidence. Understand what you might have to change about yourself and your world to reach this goal. Try to identify how you personally might affect the situation and potentially get in the way of reaching your goal. Do your negative thoughts interfere? Are there other barriers to achieving your goal, such as a controlling partner or lack of self-confidence? Find a way to work around them. Make a list of the first 3 to 5 steps to reach your goal. Try to stay focused on the goal and not on how difficult it is. Then care for yourself as you work to achieve it.

For example, if your goal is *I want to have my own opinions and control over the decisions in my life*, you might want to think of one or two examples of upcoming decisions that are important to you. Perhaps you are thinking about moving to a new place or changing jobs. Remind yourself of your reasons for wanting to do this and why it has importance and value to you. Remember that you deserve to achieve this goal. Write down the times when you made good life decisions for yourself and the result was a success.

Seek out the *facts* surrounding this decision, including, in this example, a realistic examination of your budget. What will the rent in a new apartment be? If you have a car, are there parking fees? How much will it cost to hire a moving van? Will there be additional expenses to commute to school or work? Are these items within your budget? If not, what are your concrete plans to increase your income? Can you get a part-time job? Is the grocery store, pharmacy, and laundry nearby? Think about the nonmonetary factors, such as whether you know anybody else who lives in that area. How far away do your friends and family live?

Find information online and by speaking with others about different neighborhoods in your desired town, and research possible apartment or job options. Weigh the pros and cons of this decision and think about how it will affect your life, outlining clear benefits and risks. For example, "This will help me because _____."

Think about how your own personal traits might affect your ability to make this decision, for example, are you fearful of moving to a new neighborhood or taking on a new job or financial burden? Write down the traits and concerns you have that are true and accurate in one column, and the faulty ones in another column. Think about how you might make changes in yourself to reach your goal, such as improving your tolerance of a new street or neighbors. Use your CBT skills from chapter 8 to get there.

Ask yourself if there is someone or something in your life that is preventing you from making this decision. Do you have a controlling family member, negative thoughts, or an internal fear standing in your way? If so, you will need to address those issues one by one. If you are an independent adult with a controlling parent, take steps to make your own decision without asking his or her permission to do so. You might want to wait until your decision has been made and solidified before calmly announcing your plans to your family in a strong, assertive voice. Sometimes, you have to do what is right for you regardless of the other person's inserted and unwelcome opinion. Remember that it is your life and that your opinion and desires matter.

If you have a negative thought or internal fear surrounding this decision, try the Mood and Thought Monitoring Exercise in chapter 8. This will help you uncover the distortions in your thoughts and get you on the path to achieve your goal.

Then get started. Outline the first 3 to 5 steps you must take to progress toward your goal. Identify whom you may need to assist you and help you think things through, not tell you what to do. The controlling spouse or parent is not welcome here. Try to stay focused on your desired endpoint and not on the inevitable difficulties getting there. Remember to care for yourself along the way.

Then ask yourself how this makes you feel, to make a decision free from the constraints of those people or situations who may have interfered with this in the past. Strong? Proud? Assertive? *Well* for a moment?

It is possible and realistic for those of us who have depression to expect wellness. This I know. I have lived it.

Relapse Prevention

Courage doesn't always roar. Sometimes courage is the quiet voice
at the end of the day saying, "I will try again tomorrow."
—MARY ANNE RADMACHER

OVERVIEW OF RELAPSE PREVENTION

The symptoms of major depression and bipolar disorder often fluctuate, or change up and down over time. It is important to understand that you will have fluctuations as part of the illness. The frequency and pattern of these changes will vary with each person. One way to identify your patterns is to track your symptoms on a Mood Chart (table 2.4) each day and share it with your clinician.

At some point following an episode of depression or bipolar disorder, you may have a return of symptoms, often called a recurrence or a relapse. A *relapse* is the return of full symptoms after an episode from which you have partially recovered (partial recovery means feeling improved but with a few remaining symptoms). A *recurrence* is the return of full symptoms following an episode from which you have fully recovered. Your chance of having a relapse or recurrence of depression depends in part on how many prior episodes you have had. This means that the more episodes of depression you have experienced, the greater your chance of symptoms returning at some point.

Cognitive behavioral therapy (CBT) has been shown to decrease the chance of relapse. Mindfulness-based CBT has also been shown to reduce the risk of relapse and recurrence in some patients. In addition to CBT and other psychotherapy, you can take some preventive steps to manage your own symptoms and in this way improve the quality of your life.

Relapse prevention is an effective daily approach to help you minimize the chance of a relapse occurring and to help you stay well. Relapse prevention means that you identify and respond promptly to changes in your warning signs, triggers, or symptoms of mood disorder. With this strategy, you can intervene when an important change in your emotional health may be happening. Early identification and intervention helps to prevent your episode from worsening.

A relapse prevention strategy includes five main steps that you and your treatment team will act on:

1. Identify your specific warning signs, symptoms, and triggers (see pages 106–7).
2. Pay attention to changes that are warning signs for you.
3. Prepare an intervention Action Plan for Relapse Prevention in advance for use when you notice a change in your symptoms or warning signs. The Action Plan includes steps you will take to manage, cope, and distract from the intensity of the episode. It also includes the people you will ask to help you (health care providers, family, and friends). See pages 105 and 108–15.
4. Follow your Action Plan when you first notice a change in your emotional health. An Action Plan enables you to intervene early when necessary and modify or improve the course of the episode.
5. Relapse prevention also means that you follow some basic *preventive steps* every day. These will help you maintain emotional stability and decrease your vulnerability to fluctuations, although they may not eliminate these changes completely.

Preventive steps include:

- Maintain good sleep hygiene (see pages 10–12).
- Eat three meals per day with balanced nutrition. Eat real food; avoid processed foods.
- Exercise regularly.
- Keep up with self-care.
- Maintain regular social supports and contacts.
- Avoid isolation.
- Include positive, pleasurable experiences in your life (pages 34, 126, 132, and 133).
- Keep a structure and routine to your day. Schedule your time (pages 33–34 and 38–39).
- Use your coping skills, the actions you take to lessen the effect of stressors (pages 134–38 and 157).
- Remain on your medications as prescribed.
- Do not use alcohol or drugs.
- Continue to work with your therapist.
- Continue to work on any exercises your therapist gives you.

Relapse prevention for bipolar disorder is very similar. In addition to the recommendations outlined above, a few additional tips are especially helpful to follow:

- Keep your life routine, balanced, and structured.
- Simplify your life as much as possible.
- Avoid overstimulation.
- Pace yourself, breaking large tasks down into several smaller ones.
- Find sources of replenishment and take periodic breaks in the day.
- Decrease chaotic or stimulating input at the end of the day (try relaxing, meditation, writing in your journal, taking a bath).
- Avoid impulsive actions. Wait at least two days before making any major decision or purchase, and ask two trusted friends for their feedback (the 2-Day, 2-Person Rule).
- Try social rhythm therapy, which has been formally evaluated as an intervention for bipolar disorder. It can help you keep routine and structure in your day.

AN ACTION PLAN FOR RELAPSE PREVENTION

The intervention Action Plan for Relapse Prevention outlines the steps you will take to manage, cope with, and distract from the intensity of an episode of depression or mania. It also lists the people you will ask to help you: health care providers, family, and friends. Research has shown that having a written self-care plan for situations that would lead to a worsening or a recurrence of depression can help manage depression and decrease symptoms. Work with your therapist to develop an intervention Action Plan to use when you or others notice your warning signs or a change in your emotional state.

The Action Plan includes the following elements:

- A description of your baseline
- A list of your triggers
- A list of your warning signs
- What to do in response to those warning signs
- Names and contact information for your health care providers and supportive family and friends
- Useful coping strategies
- Suggestions for how others can help

Create your Action Plan now, before you have any intense symptoms, so that you have it ready to use when you or someone else notices your warning signs.

Following is a sample Action Plan for Relapse Prevention (table 7.1) already filled out to give you an idea of its range of possibilities and how it can be used. Following that you will find a blank form to use for your own care (table 7.2).

TRIGGERS

Triggers are events or circumstances that may cause you distress and lead to an increase in your depression symptoms. It is important to understand that certain circumstances in your life have the potential to set off an episode of depression for you. Triggers can be different for each person, so to be aware of them in your everyday life, you have to first identify them for yourself.

Triggers may include such things as

- external events, good or bad
- a sudden change in your life, such as a loss (of a loved one, job, home, etc.)
- change in a relationship, or a new relationship
- change in daily routine that interrupts familiar patterns (change in sleep, meals, or activities), including around holidays and vacation times
- physical illness
- change in medications
- anniversary dates
- traumatic news or event
- good news
- feelings of stress
- feeling overwhelmed
- rejection or criticism (real or perceived)
- embarrassment or guilt
- too many or unwanted responsibilities, obligations, or tasks to do
- change of seasons

Once you have identified what events are triggers for you, you can figure out with your therapist what steps you can take to minimize their effect on you and improve the situation. You may not be able to change the trigger, but you can change your response to it. Write your triggers and these steps in your Action Plan.

Some triggers for me are

_____

_____

_____

_____

WARNING SIGNS

Warning signs are distinct changes from your baseline that precede an episode of depression or mania. Each person has a characteristic pattern of warning signs. Early recognition of yours gives you a chance to intervene and modify (change or improve) the course of the episode.

Warning signs may be a noticeable (to you or others) change in your

- thoughts
- feelings
- behaviors
- routine
- self-care

Some examples include a change from your baseline to

- having more negative thoughts
- having problems making decisions, concentrating, solving problems
- feeling more hopeless, worthless, sad, irritable, agitated, anxious, fatigued
- experiencing a lack of energy or interest, a loss of appetite, too much or too little sleep
- having difficulty getting up, going to work, shopping, maintaining your household, handling family responsibilities
- having difficulty preparing meals, eating (too much or too little), maintaining good personal hygiene, doing laundry, handling personal responsibilities

Once you have identified your warning signs, work with your therapist to determine the steps you can take to minimize or prevent the episode of depression or mania. Write these steps out in detail in your Action Plan.

Some warning signs for me are

_____

_____

_____

_____

TABLE 7.1. Sample Completed Action Plan for Relapse Prevention

MY BASELINE

Describe your baseline and what you need to do to maintain it.

When I'm feeling well, I

    get up and get showered and dressed every day

    go to work and interact with my colleagues

    go grocery shopping and prepare my meals

    exercise after work and on the weekends—aerobics, jogging, swimming, bicycling, hiking

    watch funny movies, read mystery novels, knit

    visit with my friends

To stay well, every day I need to

    take my medications

    sleep 7 hours

    eat 3 meals a day

    get exercise 5 days a week

    see my friends and family or talk to them on the phone

    keep up a routine and structure every day

MY TRIGGERS

List events and situations that can increase your symptoms.

My father calling up and criticizing me

My boss demanding that I work late

Not getting enough sleep

MY WARNING SIGNS

List your personal signs, the noticeable changes in thoughts,
feelings, behaviors, routine, or self-care that warn of an episode.

Too little sleep

Skipping meals

Avoiding friends and family

Not getting dressed or showered

Not returning phone calls

Not exercising or going out

Talking too fast

Signature (patient): _____ Date: _____

Signature (provider): _____ Date: _____

(continued)

TABLE 7.1. Sample Completed Action Plan for Relapse Prevention

WHAT I WILL DO FIRST WHEN I NOTICE MY WARNING SIGNS

☑ Contact my doctor(s) early:

Psychiatrist _Dr. Karen Smith_ _____ ph#: _____

Psychologist/therapist _Dr. Tim Jones_ _____ ph#: _____

Other _Dr. Jon Kelly_ _____ ph#: _____

☑ Treat any physical medical problems.

☑ Attend to self-care and routine, even if I don't feel like it.

☑ Get enough sleep and eat balanced meals (nutrition).

☑ Take medications as prescribed. Note any recent medication changes.

☑ NO alcohol or drugs.

☐ Other

SUPPORTIVE PERSONS I WILL CONTACT (FRIENDS, FAMILY):

1. _Sandi_ _____ ph#: _____

2. _Ginger_ _____ ph#: _____

3. _Joe_ _____ ph#: _____

4. _____ ph#: _____

5. _____ ph#: _____

WHAT I WILL DO TO COPE, SOOTHE, OR DISTRACT MYSELF:

1. *Play piano.*

2. *Listen to relaxing music.*

3. *Go to gym.*

4. *Take bubble bath.*

5. *Watch funny movies.*

WHAT I WILL *NOT* DO:

1. *Sit on couch all day.*

2. *Overeat junk food.*

3. *Not take a shower.*

HOW OTHER PEOPLE CAN HELP ME:

1. *Listen to me seriously.*

2. *Call to check on me.*

3. *Plan something to do.*

Signature (patient): _____ Date: _____

Signature (provider): _____ Date: _____

TABLE 7.2. **Action Plan for Relapse Prevention Blank Form**

MY BASELINE

Describe your baseline and what you need to do to maintain it.

When I'm feeling well, I

To stay well, every day I need to

MY TRIGGERS

List events and situations that can increase your symptoms.

MY WARNING SIGNS

*List your personal signs, the noticeable changes in thoughts,
feelings, behaviors, routine, or self-care that warn of an episode.*

Signature (patient): _____ Date: _____

Signature (provider): _____ Date: _____

(continued)

TABLE 7.2. **Action Plan for Relapse Prevention Blank Form**

WHAT I WILL DO FIRST WHEN I NOTICE MY WARNING SIGNS

☐ Contact my doctor(s) early:

Psychiatrist _____ ph#: _____

Psychologist/therapist _____ ph#: _____

Other _____ ph#: _____

☐ Treat any physical medical problems.

☐ Attend to self-care and routine, even if I don't feel like it.

☐ Get enough sleep and eat balanced meals (nutrition).

☐ Take medications as prescribed. Note any recent medication changes.

☐ NO alcohol or drugs.

☐ Other

SUPPORTIVE PERSONS I WILL CONTACT (FRIENDS, FAMILY):

1. _____ ph#: _____

2. _____ ph#: _____

3. _____ ph#: _____

4. _____ ph#: _____

5. _____ ph#: _____

WHAT I WILL DO TO COPE, SOOTHE, OR DISTRACT MYSELF:

1.

2.

3.

4.

5.

WHAT I WILL *NOT* DO:

1.

2.

3.

HOW OTHER PEOPLE CAN HELP ME:

1.

2.

3.

Signature (patient): _____ Date: _____

Signature (provider): _____ Date: _____

WHAT IF I FEEL SUICIDAL?

It's pretty common in those who have depression that a person feels alone, hopeless, and worthless and has distorted, disorganized, and negative thoughts. This may sometimes lead a person to wonder if others would be better off if she were gone, not a burden. You might not want to be around anymore. Or you could have a very specific thought of suicide, with plans for your death.

While thoughts of suicide may seem very real and urgent, don't believe them or act on them. Suicidal thoughts are wayward thoughts, not facts, and will last only a short time. Although driven by strong urges, they *will* change and go away.

Suicidal thoughts and acts happen when your deep emotional pain exceeds your ability to cope with that pain. In the chaos and anguish of the moment, it is often not possible to reach the logical part of your brain to change (or restructure) these distorted thoughts with CBT and the Mood and Thought Monitoring Exercise (described in chapter 8). It's not that you lack other solutions to your pain; it's that you *currently* are unable to see these solutions.

So, what to do? First, try to recognize that this is the depression driving your thoughts. In your baseline healthy state, suicide would not be your desire. How you feel right now is not the same as how you might feel tomorrow or next week. But this is nearly impossible to recognize in the moment. So, you need to reach out to someone you trust to help you get through this moment.

Second, suicidal thoughts are usually short lived, not permanent. Emotions are not fixed; they are constantly changing, even if you seem to return to the same familiar ones. This means that in time, they will pass. This I know firsthand. The challenge is to get yourself through this time safely, until your temporarily disorganized mind is able to manage your problems. Do whatever is necessary to get there. Recruit loved ones and your personal

> Suicide is a tragic consequence of the thought disturbances of a mood disorder. It is usually considered an impulsive act in a troubled person who sees no way to change his or her very painful circumstances. If you are feeling suicidal or in danger of harming yourself, call 1-800-273-8255 in the United States, the Samaritans in the UK or Ireland, or your local emergency number.

reasons, no matter how small, that motivate you to stay around. Once the urgency passes, you will have time to work on the problems that brought you to this point.

Pick up the phone and make a call to one of the following resources:

- A trusted family member or close friend
- Your therapist, psychiatrist, family doctor or PCP, or school counselor
- In the USA: the National Suicide Prevention Lifeline at 1-800-273-8255
- In the UK and Ireland: the Samaritans at 116 123
- In Australia: Lifeline Australia at 13 11 14
- In other countries: a local helpline listed on www.suicide.org

If you can't wait, call 9-1-1 or go to your local Emergency Department. In addition to reaching out to someone, follow these critical steps:

- Promise not to do anything right now.
- Avoid drugs and alcohol.
- Follow your safety plan, such as the Action Plan for Relapse Prevention.
- Remember those in your life who love you and would feel grief and anguish in your absence.
- Don't isolate yourself.

Sometimes having suicidal thoughts or desires means you have to be admitted to the hospital. That's okay. It might be scary at first, but just tell yourself that the hospital staff is there to help you through this. In the hospital, it feels good to be in a safe place where you will be evaluated and cared for by mental health professionals. They will offer a treatment plan, or modifications to your current plan. You still have a choice in your treatment. Soon, the urgency will pass, and you will begin to feel like yourself again.

8

Cognitive Behavioral Therapy

There is Hope because . . . we see you in a different way than you
see yourself, and if you were to see yourself as we see you,
then you could believe and hope that life could be different.
—JONATHAN E. ALPERT

THOUGHTS, FEELINGS, AND BEHAVIORS

There is a close connection between our thoughts, feelings, and behaviors (actions). Each of these influences the others. For example, a certain thought may cause you to feel sad. This may then affect your behavior, causing you to cry and withdraw. You then feel more sad. Another thought may cause you to feel anxious, and consequently your behavior is jittery.

Cognitive behavioral therapy (CBT) is a kind of talk therapy (psychotherapy) that addresses this connection between your thoughts, feelings, and behaviors. In CBT you learn to identify and change thinking patterns that may be distorted, beliefs that are inaccurate, and behaviors that are unhelpful. CBT is a way to help you look at your thoughts and determine when you are thinking in a rational or an irrational way. You learn to monitor, challenge, and replace your negative thoughts with more realistic ones and to recognize the connection between your thoughts, feelings, and behaviors.

CBT is particularly useful in depression, when your thoughts are often distorted, negative, and upsetting. If you can learn to be more aware of negative thoughts and feelings and respond to them using CBT, then you may be able to avoid a relapse or recurrence of your depression.

HOW YOU *THINK* ABOUT THE WORLD AFFECTS HOW YOU *FEEL*

- People experience the world as a series of events. These events can be positive, negative, or neutral.
- In your mind, you process and *interpret* these events and form thoughts about them. Interpretations are often based on individual beliefs and past experiences.
- Your thoughts give meaning to the event and create feelings about it.
- Feelings are created by your thoughts and interpretations of an event and not by the actual event. Thoughts and feelings are not facts.

An event can cause distress depending on how you interpret it. We often interpret events based on individual beliefs, past experiences, and our understanding of a situation. When you have an *accurate* understanding and interpretation of what is going on around you, your emotions will likely be in a normal range and not usually cause problems. If your thoughts about or interpretations of an event are inaccurate or distorted in some way, the emotions you experience may cause distress. This happens in depression. Challenging these distorted thoughts and interpretations with CBT can improve the way you feel.

What Are Thought Distortions?

Distortions in your thoughts are errors in thinking that twist your interpretation of an event in different ways (see the examples in the next section). Many things can make you less accurate in your thinking and interpretation of events, contributing to thought distortions. For example, your thinking can be affected by

- lack of sleep
- poor or imbalanced diet
- substance abuse
- past experiences
- ideas about yourself and the world (your sense of self-worth)
- your mood (such as depression or anxiety)

Thought Distortions in Depression

Depression often causes people to view their experiences, themselves, and their future in a negative way. Negative events are often magnified, dominating your thinking. The depressed mind tends to interpret and twist things in a negative direction, causing negative thoughts. These thoughts happen automatically, not on purpose.

When depressed, you are more likely to believe the biased or distorted thoughts, even though they are not an accurate reflection of reality. There is often little or no evidence to support them, and they are often extreme. But these interpretations seem true and convincing when you're in the midst of depression.

Some examples of automatic negative thoughts are

- "I'm a loser."
- "I can't do anything right."
- "Nothing is ever going to change."

These examples are extreme generalizations that are not true. Each statement is the depression talking. When you remove the distortion in these thoughts and take a more accurate view of them, you can then replace the distorted thoughts with more accurate, alternative thoughts, such as

- "I'm not perfect, but I do some things right."
- "Some things in my life do get better."

So when you are depressed, it is important to look at whether your thoughts are distorted in some way (see pages 118–20). The way to do this is to look carefully at the facts of a situation and challenge any inaccurate interpretations of them. When the distorted thought is replaced with an accurate one, the upsetting emotion will eventually be replaced by a more realistic emotion.

This is not easy to do, especially during an episode of depression, when you are viewing the world through a seemingly believable but distorted lens. You may not be able to notice the inaccuracies in your thoughts, which seem so convincing. Box 8.1 shows you how to identify the different types of distortions in your thinking and how you can learn to challenge them.

Cognitive behavioral therapy uses a series of exercises to challenge and replace the negative and distorted thoughts that accompany depression. The CBT Mood and Thought Monitoring Exercise on pages 127–28 is an effective tool for identifying the automatic distortions in your thoughts that support feelings of distress. When you practice doing this exercise, you can learn to more easily replace the distorted thought with a more accurate, realistic view. This will in turn decrease your level of distress. If this exercise is too difficult for you to do right now, at least try to remind yourself that you are depressed and that your thoughts may not be accurate at this time.

BOX 8.1. Types of Distorted Thinking

Distortions in thinking, called *cognitive distortions*, are common in depression. A person's perception or interpretation of an event can be distorted, twisted, or inaccurate in many different ways.

Filtering: focusing on and magnifying the negative details while ignoring (filtering out) all the positive aspects of a situation. When you filter your thoughts, you often reject or minimize positive experiences and insist they "don't count." Dwelling on the negative distorts your view of reality.

Polarized, or all-or-nothing, thinking: thinking of things at one extreme or the other, in black-and-white, good-or-bad, all-or-nothing categories. For example, if something you do is not perfect, you see yourself as a "total" failure, at the worst extreme.

Overgeneralizing: making a general conclusion based on a single event or piece of evidence. When you overgeneralize, you see single negative events as permanent and often use the words "always" and "never." If something bad happens, you expect it to happen again.

Global labeling: generalizing one or two qualities into a negative overall (global) judgment and applying a label. This is an extreme form of overgeneralization. An example is when you label yourself a "loser" based on one less-than-perfect behavior.

Jumping to conclusions: immediately interpreting things in a negative way without having the facts to support your conclusion.

Mind reading: concluding that you "know" what others are feeling, why they act a certain way, or how they feel about you, without their saying so.

Fortune telling: believing you "know" how future things will turn out without any supporting evidence.

Catastrophizing: expecting the worst, a disaster. This type of thinking often includes "What if" scenarios.

Minimizing: discounting the positive aspects of yourself or your actions, insisting they "don't count."

Personalizing: thinking that everything people say or do is a reaction to you personally or assuming total responsibility and blaming yourself for events out of your control.

Blaming: holding other people responsible for your pain, or the opposite, blaming yourself as the source of every problem.

Emotional reasoning: believing that what you feel *must* automatically be true, that negative emotions reflect the true picture. For example, if you *feel* stupid, then you must *be* stupid.

Being right: being continually on trial and defensive, having to prove that your feelings, opinions, and actions are right. Being wrong is unthinkable. When you think in this way, you will do anything to prove yourself right.

Reward fallacy: expecting that all your sacrifice and self-denial will pay off, then feeling bitter and resentful when that does not happen.

Source: Adapted in part from David Burns, *Feeling Good: The New Mood Therapy* (New York: Avon, 1980), table 3.1, pp. 42–43.

HOW YOU *THINK* AND *FEEL* ALSO AFFECTS HOW YOU *ACT*

Your interpretations of the events in your life cause emotions, and in response to these emotions, you have an urge to act in a certain way. For example, when feeling sad and miserable, you may choose to act angrily, stay in bed, cry, or drink too much alcohol. While some expression of emotion is okay, these are extreme negative behaviors that are not healthy for you.

Since you have the ability to act on your feelings, you also have *some* control over your emotions by choosing *how* to react and respond to them. The actions and decisions you make in response can intensify or lessen a particular feeling. Learning to modify your responses to intense emotion will decrease your level of distress. For example, instead of feeling extremely "enraged" or out of control in response to a troubling situation, you might feel sad or moderately angry. Work with your therapist to learn and practice this skill.

SHOULD STATEMENTS

Should statements are things you say that start off with the words "I should." They reflect a rigid set of rules about how you and others must act, think, or feel. These statements take a *desire* and change it to a mandatory inflexible standard, a moral imperative. When applied to the past, you can never meet that standard of perfection, so you end up feeling guilty, frustrated, or angry.

For example, "I should have done _____" reflects a situation that can never be met.

Be aware of the "musts," "oughts," "shoulds," and any "standards" you have that others do not share.

Ways to handle should statements:

1. Recognize the standards you cannot reach.
2. Recognize these statements as *desires*, not mandatory rules.
3. Replace thinking "I should _____" with
   "*I wish I* _____," or
   "*I would like* _____."
4. Practice doing this exercise when you catch yourself using a should statement.

CHALLENGING AND CHANGING YOUR THOUGHTS

Mood and Thought Monitoring Exercise

The Mood and Thought Monitoring Exercise is an effective CBT tool used to monitor and modify the negative thoughts and emotions that come with depression. In this exercise you will

- look at a particular situation that caused you to feel distress,
- identify the distortions in the thoughts that support those feelings of distress,
- challenge the negative, distorted thoughts, and
- replace them with a more accurate view.

This process, called *cognitive restructuring*, has been found to improve current levels of distress in people struggling with depression. The Mood and Thought Monitoring Exercise is an effective tool to use with your therapist or treatment team. The technique was originally presented by Aaron T. Beck as the "Daily Record of Dysfunctional Thoughts." It has also been described in detail by David Burns in his book *Feeling Good*. The exercise has been widely used clinically and adapted by many others since then. See box 8.2 for additional ways to challenge your thinking and therefore improve your mood.

Purpose of the Mood and Thought Monitoring Exercise

1. Self-assessment
   - To increase your awareness of your thoughts, emotions, feelings, reactions, interpretations
   - To understand how your thoughts, feelings, and actions (behaviors) are related and how they affect each other
   - To understand what events led up to your current feelings

2. Changing your problematic thinking
   - Identify the thoughts that come automatically and support bad feelings (*automatic negative thoughts*), then replace them with a more accurate view of the situation.
   - Identify ways to think differently about yourself and a situation, increase your awareness and perspective, and gain objectivity. Correct errors in your thinking.

How to Use the Mood and Thought Monitoring Exercise

Pick a recent personal experience to think about. Fill in the five columns from left to right on the Mood and Thought Monitoring Exercise form (see table 8.1). Then reflect on your thoughts and emotions about the experience. This is not an easy task to do, and it may stir up the emotions you are now thinking about. Review the completed monitoring form with your therapist. Doing this exercise regularly will change your emotions in general and those related to each experience in particular. It will eventually improve your mood.

Fill in the Mood and Thought Monitoring Exercise form with your responses to these five steps.

1. Choose a recent situation or event that triggered distressed feelings in you and that is associated with one or more automatic negative thoughts.
2. Notice the emotions associated with that situation (such as sadness, anxiety, fear).
3. Identify the automatic negative thought(s) raised by that situation.
4. Identify the distortions in your thoughts (see Types of Distorted Thinking, on page 121). Replace the distorted, inaccurate thought with a realistic *alternative thought* (this is called a *rational response*). The alternative thought you choose must be a fair and more accurate view of the situation. It has to be realistic, honest, and believable, and it should validate the emotion you are experiencing.
5. Notice the change in your emotions or in their intensity after you have replaced your thoughts with a more accurate, realistic view.

Example Responses to the Mood and Thought Monitoring Exercise

A situation that triggered thoughts: John did not return my telephone call when he said he would.

Emotions associated with this situation: sadness, anger, rejection—at 100 percent intensity.

Automatic negative thoughts: He hates me. He is angry with me. Everybody hates me. I'm a loser. I did something wrong. I'm not important enough.

Distortions in those thoughts: polarized thinking, overgeneralization, mind reading, catastrophizing.

Alternative thought: John is my long-time friend, and he has never given
  me reason to think he hates me. There is no reason to think he is
  angry with me that I know of. Some people like me. I do some things
  right. There is no reason to think that I did something wrong to John.
  Maybe he is busy or out of town. Maybe he is sick or it slipped his
  mind.

Emotions after restructuring your thoughts: sadness: 10 percent intensity;
  angry: 20 percent intensity; rejected: 10 percent intensity.

Notice how the restructured alternative thought has improved the intensity of the initial emotions from 100 percent to 10–20 percent.

EVIDENCE FOR AND AGAINST

When a thought, belief, or interpretation of an event is troubling, it is often
helpful to examine the evidence for and against that thought (table 8.2). The
evidence you gather will help you identify and change thoughts that are
based on inaccurate assumptions.

Step 1. Identify a belief or thought that is negative or upsetting.

Step 2. Gather evidence for and against that thought.

- Collect specific evidence about that thought to check its accuracy.
- Ask others who know you well for their realistic, honest feedback
  about that thought.
- Seek out experiences that counteract your negative beliefs. This
  means that you go out and do something to see firsthand the evidence against your negative belief.

Step 3. Look at your list realistically and see where the evidence lies.

Ask yourself if your belief is inherently true or if it is an internalized
message from your environment. If you find it is true, ask yourself, what is
in your power to change?

Here's an example of how you might use this exercise. Imagine for a
moment that you have the following thought: *I'm no good at socializing and
making friends*. In Step 2 you would think about the recent and past times
you made a connection with someone else that felt good. List them in the
column "Evidence against it" on table 8.2. For example, "I made a new friend,
Jeff, through my photography class." Then list any specific examples of "Evidence for" that thought in the middle column. If you have trouble doing this,
ask someone whose opinion you trust to help you, such as a relative. Next,

go out and test your belief in the real world—attend an event and note the times you were or were not able to connect with another person.

In Step 3 you would sit down and look at how you filled out your form and truly think about the evidence you gathered in each column. Ask yourself what is true and what thought is a hidden message from your upbringing or your environment. If you find a thought with evidence indicating that it is true, ask yourself what in your life you can change.

Another useful exercise is to try understanding where a particular thought comes from, its origin. Perhaps a certain thought that bothers you began in childhood or adolescence and stems from an unpleasant experience that no longer applies to your current life. It might be something a parent, teacher, or friend said or did that still plagues you now. Sometimes these thoughts stick with you for years, haunting you and causing distress. Spending time reacting to old thoughts that no longer apply is not helpful in the present. Table 8.3 provides one way to help you identify when this is going on.

PLEASURE AND MASTERY

Add some pleasure and mastery activities to your week, even if you don't feel like it or don't feel that you deserve it. Eliminating negative experiences from your life is not enough. You also need to have positive and pleasurable experiences. Pleasurable activities will help decrease the chance of your depressive symptoms getting worse. Table 8.4 lists examples of pleasurable activities. They are a way to help yourself, part of your relapse prevention plan.

Create a list of pleasurable activities that you like to do, or used to like to do. Choose to do some of these regularly, and add them to your daily schedule (table 8.5).

Next, list activities you like that challenge you, that provide you with a feeling of competence and effectiveness. They should be a little difficult for you to do (such as overcoming an obstacle or learning a new skill). These are called mastery activities. Choose to do some of these on a regular basis, and add them to your schedule. Examples include improving your time while jogging, learning a new language, mastering a new application on your computer, or overcoming a fear of something by doing it in small steps.

TABLE 8.1. **Mood and Thought Monitoring Exercise**

Use this form to monitor your mood when you are feeling unpleasant emotion or distress. The purpose is to identify the thoughts you have that support or contribute to the distressed feelings and to help you develop a more accurate view of the situation. Review the completed form with your therapist or treatment team.

SITUATION	EMOTION	AUTOMATIC THOUGHT
Describe an event, thought, or memory that triggers unpleasant emotions or distress.	Record your current emotions and rate the intensity from 0 to 100 (e.g., anxious, angry, sad, guilty, ashamed).	Record the associated thoughts you are having that intensify your emotions.

(*continued*)

TABLE 8.1. Mood and Thought Monitoring Exercise

ALTERNATIVE (RATIONAL) RESPONSE	EMOTIONS AFTER RATIONAL RESPONSE
Identify the distortions in your thoughts. Rewrite the distorted thought as a statement with a fair and more accurate view of the situation.	Record your emotion(s) again and rerate the intensity, 0 to 100.

Source: Adapted with permission from Aaron T. Beck, A. John Rush, Brian F. Shaw, and Gary Emery, *Cognitive Therapy of Depression* (New York: Guilford Press, 1979), 403.

BOX 8.2. More Ways to Challenge and Change Your Thinking

- Identify the distortions in your thinking. Use the Types of Distorted Thinking descriptions on page 121 as a guide.

- Use the CBT Mood and Thought Monitoring Exercise to evaluate a situation associated with emotional distress. Substitute a more realistic thought or interpretation of an event for your distorted one.

- Examine the Evidence For and Against a negative thought, belief, or interpretation of an event.

  – Gather evidence.

    · Conduct your own "experiment" and gather evidence to check the accuracy of your thought.

    · Ask others who know you well for their realistic, honest feedback.

    · Seek out experiences that counteract the negative beliefs you have.

  – Ask if your belief is inherently true or if it is an internalized message from your environment.

    – If it is true, what is in your power to change?

- Examine the pros and cons of any thought, belief, decision, or action.

- When a thought or belief is upsetting you, look at whether your thought and reaction have more to do with events from long ago. Ask yourself:

  – Where does this thought come from?

  – Does it apply *now*, in the current situation?

- Separate your opinion and interpretation from fact. Interpretations often distort a situation negatively.

- Avoid making judgments or interpretations. Feelings and interpretations are not facts.

  – Rely on the facts. Ask yourself: Is this an interpretation, or is it a *fact*?

- Replace should statements with less demanding language, such as "I would like it if . . ."

- Instead of assuming full responsibility and blame for a particular problem, consider other factors that might have contributed, that were outside your control.

- Use the same compassion in talking to yourself as you would give to others.

- Try thinking of things in the middle ground, or gray area, instead of at the extremes of black and white.

TABLE 8.2. Evidence For and Against		
BELIEF OR THOUGHT	EVIDENCE FOR IT	EVIDENCE AGAINST IT

TABLE 8.3. Understanding the Origins of Your Thoughts

Sometimes the thoughts that bother us come from situations long ago, but the thoughts stay with us, even though they no longer apply. Spending time reacting to old thoughts does not help your current situation.

Ask whether your distressed thought or reaction applies to the current situation or to events in your past. Does it apply now? If it does not apply now, try to put it aside.

DISTRESSED THOUGHT OR REACTION	WHERE DOES THAT COME FROM?	DOES IT APPLY NOW?

TABLE 8.4. **Examples of Pleasurable Activities**

We each have our own preferences for pleasurable activities. Here are some examples:

Relax (on your own or using a relaxation tape)
Stretch
Get physical exercise
Go for a walk outdoors
Enjoy the weather
Bicycle
Garden
Play a sport
Watch sports
Listen to music
Attend a concert
Play an instrument
Sing
Learn a new language
Look at beautiful scenery
Look at beautiful art
Go to a museum
Enjoy a good fragrance or other smell
Indulge in self-care (bubble bath, etc.)
Get a massage
Get your hair done
Have a manicure or pedicure
Cook
Eat a good meal
Go on a date
Enjoy quiet time
Play a game

Spend time with friends
Spend time with family you enjoy
Spend time with children
Volunteer
Do a jigsaw puzzle
Do Sudoku
Do a crossword puzzle
Play with a pet
Meditate
Work on a favorite project
Learn something new
Reach a goal
Travel
Work on a favorite hobby
Read a good book or magazine
Read the comics
Plan a party
Go to a party
Give someone a gift
Watch a good or funny movie
Laugh
Shop or window shop
Knit, crochet, do needlepoint
Do woodworking, other crafts
Build something
And lots of other things . . .

What is pleasurable for me?

TABLE 8.5. **Pleasure and Mastery Exercise**

PLEASURE ACTIVITIES
Things I like (or used to like) to do:

MASTERY ACTIVITIES
Things I like (or used to like) to do that challenge me
and give a sense of competence and accomplishment:

9

Strategies to Get You through the Tough Times

*The greatest weapon against stress is our ability to choose
one thought [or action] over another.*
—WILLIAM JAMES

The life skills described in this chapter can help you through some of the rough times. A few of the approaches are a review from previous chapters, included here as a reminder because they can be difficult to remember and do when depressed. You will learn strategies for coping and stress, mindfulness, and distress tolerance. In addition, there is an overview of communication skills, with recommendations for talking with your doctor and tips you can suggest to family and friends.

COPING AND STRESS

Stress is an emotionally and physically disturbing condition you may have in response to challenging life events. When you are suffering from depression, dealing with stress can be more difficult. It can also make your depression worse and contribute to relapse (a return of symptoms).

Stress can come from events inside or outside you. The causes and intensity of stress may vary from person to person, but common causes include:

- real events in life (positive or negative, e.g., marriage, divorce, birth, job, finances, a major loss)
- relationships
- an illness
- change (of any kind)
- your environment
- overload of responsibilities

- an unresolved conflict
- a situation not under your control
- uncertainty while waiting on an unknown outcome

You can actively take steps to lessen the effects of stress and decrease your vulnerability to stressors. This is called *coping*. When you manage stress using effective coping strategies, you decrease the negative effect that stress has on your depression. Box 9.1 lists examples of coping strategies.

Coping strategies include ways to prevent and prepare for stress as well as skills for managing it when it occurs:

1. Maintain a regular schedule and structure of activities. This includes optimizing your sleep, diet and nutrition, exercise, and self-care.
2. Manage the little daily stressors.
   - Prioritize your responsibilities and activities.
   - Keep yourself organized.
   - Maintain a schedule but don't overschedule, and adjust as needed.
   - Break down large or complex tasks into smaller pieces that are more manageable.
   - Keep a to-do list and a daily reminders list.
   - Write things down in a notebook, including health care–related questions and instructions.
   - Use a daily pillbox for your medications, to keep track of when you took them.
   - Develop a system that you like and that works for you to manage the mail, bills, and housekeeping.
   - Avoid overstimulation.
   - Be mindful, in this moment.
3. Use CBT strategies. An event can cause stress depending on how you interpret it. Usually we interpret events based on individual beliefs and past experiences. Sometimes we also interpret events with distortions in our thinking. Challenging these distorted thoughts and interpretations using cognitive behavioral therapy can affect the way you feel and respond and can improve your level of stress.
   - Use the CBT exercises (see chapter 8).
   - Keep a journal of your thoughts and feelings.
   - Identify the sources of your stress. This will help you respond to it in a more effective way, when you know what you are dealing with.
   - Be assertive in your communication—this helps you feel in control of your situation.
   - Keep your perspective.

4. Use problem-solving strategies.
   - Speak with someone (a friend, therapist) for help as you work out a problem.
   - Get accurate information about the problem to make an informed decision.
   - Evaluate and define the situation realistically.
   - Consider your options and the alternatives.
   - List the pros and cons of your options.
   - Seek additional assistance as needed.

5. Distract and refocus your attention.
   - Occupy your mind with other thoughts and activities: puzzles, reading, hobbies, sports, gardening, or other things you like to do.
   - Volunteer your time; reach out to others.
   - Replace your current emotion with another (e.g., by watching a movie or reading a book that is funny or scary).
   - Leave the situation aside mentally for a while.

6. Try relaxation techniques (work with your therapist to learn these skills).
   - Progressive muscle relaxation—relax each muscle in your body from head to toe, one muscle group at a time (start with your jaw, then move to your neck, shoulders, arms, fingers, etc.).
   - Visualization—sit and focus on a calm, serene image or a place where you feel relaxed.
   - Biofeedback—discuss with your therapist how to learn this technique.
   - Meditation—Herbert Benson's book *The Relaxation Response* gives detailed information on getting started.
   - Deep breathing exercise—sit quietly and focus only on your breathing, taking slow deep breaths. Do this for 3 to 5 minutes. If your mind wanders, refocus on each breath.

7. Use humor: watch a funny movie on Netflix or DVD, read a funny book or the comics. Being able to appreciate humor is a healthy coping strategy.

8. Use self-soothing strategies—comfort and nurture yourself with gentleness and kindness, using the five senses.
   - *Vision:* enjoy looking at flowers, art, or other objects of beauty; visit museums; get out in nature; see a play, musical, or dance production.
   - *Taste:* enjoy a favorite food or beverage; take it slow and savor the experience.

- *Smell:* use a favorite fragrance or lotion; buy flowers or walk through a flower garden or shop; bake cinnamon rolls or cookies.
- *Touch:* take a bubble bath, get a massage, wear comfortable fabrics, hug someone.
- *Hearing:* listen to beautiful, soothing music or sounds of nature; sing; play an instrument.
9. Use mindfulness techniques (see below).
   - Focus on the present moment, on purpose, nonjudgmentally.
   - Focus on doing one thing at a time, in just this moment.
   - Avoid ruminating about the past or worrying about the future.

MINDFULNESS

Mindfulness is a way of living your life by focusing on the present moment. It is a way of "being" in the world, adopted from Eastern meditation practices. The skills learned in mindfulness practice have been found helpful in managing mood disorders.

As described by Jon Kabat-Zinn, mindfulness means being in the present moment in a particular way by

- paying attention
- on purpose
- nonjudgmentally

Being in the present moment means that instead of being preoccupied with the past or future, you are focused on and attentive to the present. This is not easy to do. It is common for the mind to wander, particularly to thoughts of past events or future worries. The key is to notice when your thoughts drift and then bring your mind back to the present. Becoming so deeply involved in doing something that you lose track of time is an example of being in the present moment.

Mindfulness requires that you *pay attention* to what is going on around you. It means that you live with awareness instead of going through life on autopilot. Paying attention also involves observing your own thoughts and feelings, your body's response to emotion (such as rapid heart rate, sweating, etc.), your urges, and your behavior just as they are.

Being *nonjudgmental* means that you avoid making any judgment about your thoughts, actions, or experiences and let each moment be as it is. Allow yourself to think or feel what you are feeling, without putting labels or judgment on it. This is also not easy to do. Part of your mind is constantly evaluating your experiences, comparing them to past experiences or expectations you may have. Instead, work on developing a neutral attitude toward what comes into your mind without judging it. Acknowledge your thoughts as thoughts and then let them go. For each experience, emotion, or thought you have, try to feel it without reacting to it. Here's one way to try it. Imagine yourself sitting in a car on a foggy day, with the windshield wipers going

---

BOX 9.1. Coping Strategies

Try any of these examples of coping strategies to find what works for you. The more familiar you are with your options, the easier it will be to remember them during stressful times or an episode of depression or mania.

- Ask for help.
- Don't give up.
- Do the best with what you have available to you now.
- Focus on what matters.
- Seek a solution to the problem.
- Seek out the facts. Identify and challenge any inaccurate assumptions and interpretations.
- List your options.
- Examine the evidence for and against.
- Try an alternative approach, a different way of thinking.
- Anticipate, think, and plan ahead.
- Be active, not passive.
- Be assertive.
- Listen to your needs.
- Say no when necessary.
- Get organized.
- Control what you can.
- Set realistic and specific goals.

- Balance and prioritize.
- Pace yourself.
- Don't overcommit.
- Structure your day.
- Take good care of your body (sleep, diet, exercise).
- Treat yourself with compassion and respect.
- Focus on the present moment.
- Use self-soothing.
- Give yourself credit.
- Reward yourself.
- Stay safe. Avoid situations that could worsen your symptoms.
- Consider the consequences of your actions and decisions.
- Watch for your triggers and warning signs. Activate your Action Plan for Relapse Prevention as needed.
- Develop some distress tolerance (using distraction, self-soothing, improving the moment; see pages 97 and 140–42).

slowly. Each stray thought is like a leaf that lands on the windshield. Allow the wiper blades to brush the leaf (thought) away with one or two strokes of the blade, letting it go.

Why Practice Mindfulness?

- Living mindfully allows you to engage in what you are doing. Emotions will interfere less often. This will improve the quality of your life.
- Mindfulness helps you to live in the present moment instead of experiencing painful emotions related to the past or future. Dwelling on past experiences or future worries tends to trigger painful emotions. This happens often in depression. Mindfulness practice helps you to decrease these ruminations (see chapter 3) and the emotions and distress they produce.
- Mindfulness practice can help you manage your mood disorder. When you have an increased awareness of the present moment, you are able to notice when symptoms of your mood disorder arise. Recognizing your depression or bipolar symptoms enables you to respond effectively with your relapse prevention plan.
- Mindfulness can improve your ability to tolerate and respond to painful events. When you are overwhelmed by emotions, your mind clutters up quickly. So you have to focus first on the thought or moment and try to clear your mind, to calm it down. To do this you must step back, observe your own thought, and try to get a handle on it. Mindfulness practice can help you do this. When you are focused on and attentive to the present moment, without attaching judgment or value to it, you can make the best use of your thoughts, take action, and work on your problem.
- Many people find that mindfulness-based cognitive behavioral therapy is an effective treatment for depression.

How Do You Practice Mindfulness?

Mindfulness is a skill that you can develop with practice. Begin by trying to make yourself more aware of the present moment without judging it as good or bad. Focus your full attention on what you are doing, on one thing at a time. Get fully involved in that moment. Notice when your mind wanders and bring your attention back to the moment. You can begin to practice this by setting aside 5 minutes a day to do a mindfulness meditation (see below).

You can also try to exercise mindfulness as you go about your day. For example, when you brush your teeth, focus your mind on doing only that one task. Pay attention to your actions, to the taste, sensations, sounds, and so on. As your mind wanders, bring it back to the task of brushing your teeth in this moment. Try it again when you drive, wash the dishes, have a conversation, or during other moments of your life. Live with awareness of what you are doing instead of going through life automatically.

Exercise to Practice Being Mindful
1. Sit in a comfortable chair, in a comfortable position.
2. Close your eyes if you like.
3. Become aware of your breathing, and focus on each breath.
4. Anchor your attention to the present moment: pay attention to your breathing, the sounds around you, the physical sensations you have.
5. Observe what you feel, see, and hear without placing a value or judgment on it.
6. Continue to focus on each breath, in and out.
7. When intrusive thoughts come into your mind, let them go without judging them or yourself. Return your focus to your breathing. Over time it will become easier to focus your mind in this way.

DISTRESS TOLERANCE

Sometimes the intensity of depression is so deep, it feels like a crisis. You may feel a sense of urgency or a desire to act impulsively. You may feel there is no way out. These feelings can interfere with your efforts to manage depression and maintain stability. Learning to tolerate distress for a short time can help you get through a difficult moment, when you cannot change the situation. Distress tolerance strategies help you do this by using skills to distract yourself, soothe yourself, provide solace, and improve the difficult moment.

These strategies are not a cure for the problems of life. They are not meant to dismiss the seriousness of your problems. Practicing distress tolerance is more like taking a break from your situation for a short while. Use these skills when you feel overwhelmed by your depression. Eventually the intensity of the moment will fade away.

Strategies to Achieve Distress Tolerance

Distraction

Decrease your contact with events that trigger distress using:

- activities, such as hobbies, sports, or gardening, to distract your attention
- other thoughts or sensations to distract your mind (such as by doing puzzles, reading)
- contribution—reach out, volunteer, find a sense of meaning
- comparison—with those less fortunate
- emotions—replace a current emotion with another one (such as by watching a funny or scary movie)

Note: Keep in mind that short-term distraction is not the same as avoiding a problem. Don't push away—avoidance is not helpful as a regular strategy.

Self-Soothing

Be kind to yourself. Comfort and nurture yourself by engaging the five senses:

- Vision: enjoy looking at flowers, art, or other objects of beauty; visit museums; get out in nature; see a play, musical, or dance production.
- Taste: enjoy a favorite food or beverage; take it slow and savor the experience.
- Smell: use a favorite fragrance or lotion; buy flowers or walk through a flower garden or shop; bake cinnamon rolls or cookies.
- Touch: take a bubble bath, get a massage, wear comfortable fabrics, hug someone.
- Hearing: listen to beautiful, soothing music or sounds of nature; sing; play an instrument.

Note: Some people feel they are not deserving, or they feel guilt or shame when using self-soothing strategies. If these are problems for you, work on them with your therapist or treatment team.

Improving the Moment

To replace the immediate negative event with a positive experience or image, try the these techniques:

- Visualization—sit and focus on a calm, serene image or a place where you feel relaxed

- Meditation—Herbert Benson's book *The Relaxation Response* gives detailed information on getting started
- Mindfulness—focus on one thing in the moment (see the Mindfulness exercise on page 140)
- Breathing exercise—sit quietly and focus only on your breathing, taking slow deep breaths, for 3 to 5 minutes; if your mind wanders, refocus on each breath
- Prayer
- Relaxation techniques
- Encouraging self-talk (be your own cheerleader)
- Thinking of pros and cons—the positive and negative aspects of tolerating distress

Basic Principles of Distress Tolerance

- Tolerating distress requires the ability to accept yourself and the current situation.
- Acceptance does not mean you approve of the distressing situation. It is not the same as judging it as good.
- Acceptance is a skill for tolerating and surviving the crisis in the moment, until the intensity fades. It will fade.

COMMUNICATION SKILLS

With depression, speaking up and advocating for yourself can be hard to do. You may feel that your needs, feelings, or opinions are not important or deserving. But symptoms of depression can worsen if you hold things inside when you are upset and don't talk about what you want and need. This can also lower your self-esteem. It is important to communicate clearly and effectively so that the other person really *hears* you. Your style of communication determines whether and how your message is received. Communication styles can be described as *aggressive, assertive, passive,* or a combination (*passive-aggressive*).

An *aggressive* communication style is dominating, with yelling, threats, and anger. It is not effective. Aggressiveness tends to alienate other people, making them defensive. You don't accomplish what you want with this communication style, and you don't feel good about yourself. Try to avoid this style.

A *passive* style, when you remain quiet and submissive, is also not effective. When you are passive, you don't speak up to make your needs and wants known. When you do not speak up and advocate for yourself, you run the risk of doing and becoming what other people want you to do and be. Your needs and wants are not met. Other people respond in a way that is not in your best interest, and you do not accomplish your goals. You then have no control over what happens to you and often feel worse about yourself. You want to avoid being passive.

Being *assertive* means that you stand up for yourself in a calm, confident manner (box 9.2). You express your beliefs, opinions, wants, and needs effectively and do what you believe is right. With this communication style, you have a greater chance of being able to negotiate what you want and need. When you are assertive, you feel better about yourself for stating what you want, need, or feel. Self-esteem improves, and you have an increased sense of control over what happens to you. This is the preferred communication style for you.

BOX 9.2. Assertiveness

These guidelines can help you learn to communicate assertively, and therefore more effectively:

- Speak up. Believe you have the right to what you want and need.

- Be clear, concise, and firm.

- Appear confident in voice, tone, and manner.

- Use a calm, neutral voice. The tone you use can change your message (the most common tones people use are angry, nasty, meek, passive, aggressive, and neutral).

- Use neutral body language, because body position can change your message.

  - Sit up straight, with an open, relaxed posture and easy manner.

  - Make eye contact.

  - Do not cross your arms, point a finger, make a fist, or fidget.

- Express your feelings, opinions, and wishes.

- Use statements, not questions.

- Use "I" statements, such as "I would like" and "I feel."

- Do not make accusations or threats. Do not say, "You did" or "You should." That empowers other people and makes them defensive.

- Focus on your objectives and avoid straying from the topic.

(*continued*)

- It may help to plan what you will say in advance and write it down.
- Listen to other people. Try to validate and understand their positions as well.
- Ask questions to clarify what you do not understand.
- Negotiate a solution that maintains your integrity and values.
- You do not have to respond to the other person in the moment of emotion. It is okay to say, "Let me gather my thoughts and discuss this later," and then do it when you feel calmer.
- Don't expect to be always aware of or able to handle your thoughts and feelings immediately, in the midst of discussion or emotion. It's okay to respond later on by saying, "I've thought about this for a while and . . ."

An important communication skill to learn is that of effective listening. Many of us are racing forward with our own thoughts and don't hear or demonstrate that we have heard what the other person has said. This sends out a message of indifference and of not being very interested in others. Listening can help enrich our relationships. We all have room for improvement in our listening communication skills. Making direct eye contact, giving your full attention, and validating the other's experience are simple yet effective things you can do. They may be a bit more challenging when depressed and your concentration and focus are not optimal; keep trying anyway. Helpful listening skills are outlined in box 9.3, along with blocks to effective listening.

BOX 9.3. Listening

Listening is a communication skill that is important to maintaining your relationships. Everyone has room for improvement in this area. With depression, the thought distortions and lack of concentration can affect your ability to listen well and communicate clearly and effectively. Practice using these recommendations to improve your ability to listen and to relate well in your relationships.

- Make eye contact.
- Use open, neutral body language: sit up straight, with an inviting, relaxed posture.

- Give your full attention.
- Show genuine interest.
- Smile. Be relaxed and warm. Use humor.
- Validate and acknowledge the other person's experience (e.g., nod your head). Do not be dismissive, make assumptions, refer to your own personal experiences, or give advice.
- Periodically summarize what the other person says. For example:
  - "It appears that _____," "It sounds like _____," "What you seem to be saying is _____."
  - "Is that the case? Do I understand correctly?"
- Clarify the other person's points and comments.
- Offer feedback—share what you thought, felt, and sensed in the conversation without being judgmental. Be honest and supportive.

Some things can get in the way of effective listening. Be aware of times when you might make these mistakes. This awareness will help you improve your listening skills.

Blocks to effective listening include:

- Making assumptions (without the facts)
- Filtering out what the person is saying (when you avoid hearing some of the details)
- Changing the subject to yourself or another topic
- Comparing the person's experience to another experience
- Mind reading (when you conclude, without the facts, that you know what the other person is thinking)
- Rehearsing (when you focus on what you are going to say next)
- Judging what the other person is saying
- Identifying (when you refer to your own similar experience)
- Daydreaming, not paying attention
- Giving advice
- Sparring, using put-downs or sarcasm, debating a point
- Having to be right at any length
- Placating the other person

TALKING WITH YOUR DOCTOR

A good working relationship with your treatment team (psychiatrist, clinical psychologist, or therapist) is essential to managing your depression or bipolar disorder. Your treatment is a collaboration between you and your health care providers. You must be able to communicate well with each other so that your needs are understood and met. This includes taking the time to ask questions and make your concerns known.

Come prepared for your appointments by writing down in advance:

- any new problems, side effects, or issues since the last visit
- questions you would like to ask
- topics or treatments to clarify or review
- a list of current medications and dosages (include nonprescription vitamins and herbal supplements as well as information about your medication allergies and any significant adverse reactions to medications you have had)

Be sure to prioritize your issues. Understand that not everything can be covered in one session. You might find it helpful to use a small notebook for recording the above information as well as treatment instructions in detail, homework assignments, appointments, information about past medications, and so forth. To communicate effectively during the appointment, follow these guidelines:

- Speak up. Let your doctor know what issues are important to you.
- Try to be as clear, concise, and accurate as possible.
- Ask questions. For example:
  - What is wrong with me? What is my diagnosis?
  - What treatment or medications do you recommend and why?
  - Are there other treatment options?
  - What are the benefits and risks of this treatment?
  - How long will it take to know if this treatment is effective?
  - How should I expect to feel with this medication? What side effects might I have?
- When you receive instructions from your doctor, write them down in detail. It is often difficult to listen and remember complex information.
- Ask your doctor to repeat or clarify points or instructions you do not understand or remember, or that seem vague or uncertain. Do not leave the appointment if you are unclear about any instructions.

- Don't be embarrassed if you forget or do not understand something. No question is "dumb."
- Don't be concerned that your provider will be "angry" with you or will refuse to answer your question.
- People differ in the amount of information or detail they want to know about their illness. Some may want only a basic overview, while others feel more in control of what is happening to them when they know the facts. Decide what is best for you and let your doctor know.

If you have a problem communicating with your doctor, state your concern as honestly and openly as possible, in a nonthreatening manner, without making accusations. For example, you might say,

- "I'm concerned that we aren't communicating as well as we could, such as when _____."
- "I need to be able to talk with you about _____, and I feel like I can't. Can we discuss this?"
- "I would like to discuss _____ at more length. Can we schedule a time for that?"
- "I am having trouble understanding _____. Can you help me understand?"

TIPS FOR FAMILY AND FRIENDS

Your family members and close friends may often struggle with knowing how to best help you during an episode of depression. They may wonder: *What should I say? What can I do to help?* We each have our own way of coping with stressful situations and illness. We have our own set of personal experiences with illness, relationships, life events, and work. Because of these differences, people have varying needs, and there are many ways to offer help. Here are some suggestions you can pass along to them.

Do try to:

- Be present and give your full attention; have your mind "in the moment."
- Listen. This sounds simple, but it may be hard to do. You don't always have to respond. Sometimes an empathetic listener is what the person needs the most.
- Let him know that you care. Be mindful that greater patience and compassion may be called for during certain times.
- Validate the person's feelings. Make him feel he is worthwhile.

- If you want to offer encouragement, remind the person of her special qualities (like a sense of humor) and other successfully managed challenges or accomplishments.
- Know the symptoms of depression, mania, and suicide risk.
- Be aware of the person's warning signs, which precede a worsening episode of depression or mania, and know when to encourage the call for professional help.
- Respect a person's choice about how much she wants to share. Some people are very private while others will talk more about their depression. If someone confides in you, keep the conversation private. Ask how much the person wants others to know.
- If asked, be available to help the person talk through treatment decisions, but do not offer advice. Respect decisions about treatment even if you disagree.
- Offer to help with routine tasks, but do not take over. Look for ways to encourage and facilitate the person's self-care.
- Offer to help in concrete, specific ways (pick up grocery items, walk the dog, go with her to an appointment).
- Include the person in the usual activities and social events. Let him be the one to determine if something is too much to manage.
- Keep your relationship as normal and balanced as possible. The person may appreciate conversations and activities that don't involve depression.
- Expect the person to have good days and bad days, emotionally and physically.

Do *not*:

- Offer advice or be judgmental.
- Compare the person's experience to others you have known.
- Automatically offer reassuring words when someone expresses despair or a dark emotion. Before saying, "You'll be fine," think about whether you are saying this to calm your own anxiety and fear. Sometimes it can cause the person to feel dismissed rather than supported.
- Take things too personally. It's not uncommon for a person who has a mood disorder to be more quiet or irritable than usual.
- Be afraid to talk about depression or mania or to ask about suicidal thoughts.

For more ideas on how to help a loved one who has a mood disorder, check out my second book: *When Someone You Know Has Depression: Words to Say and Things to Do*. I think you'll find it helpful.

Dealing with Family and Friends

The best kind of people . . . make you see the sun where you once saw clouds. The people that believe in you so much, you start to believe in you too.
—KATE LATTEY, *AGAINST THE CLOCK*

Managing your illness and staying well is often easier when you have a good support system that can help you through difficult situations. This is the ideal, but it is not always available to everyone for many reasons. Family members or friends are not always as reliable or understanding as you'd like, or they might be busy at your moment of need. And sometimes asking for support can be scary. As described by clinical psychologist Louisa Sylvia, there are two reasons for this. You might fear being hurt by others, especially those who know you well, because you care about what they think. They know how to "push your buttons" in a disagreement.

You also might be afraid of letting others down, fearing that you can't hold up your end of the bargain in a friendship. For example, during a mood disorder episode, you might cancel plans to get together, fail to return phone calls or e-mails, and so forth. These behaviors feed into the self-doubts and feelings of worthlessness you may have.

For many people, one of the toughest, most stressful parts of having a mood disorder is discussing their illness with family and friends. Loved ones may have different viewpoints, knowledge, and understanding about mood disorders, and this can interfere with your communication and the relationship. Personal relationships surrounding your illness usually fall into three categories:

1. People you choose to tell about your mood disorder who are mainly supportive
2. People who know about it and are not supportive
3. People you choose not to tell (such as a distant acquaintance or an employer)

Most individuals with mood disorders have a variety of these relationships to manage, and you are not alone if you feel that a family member does not understand your illness or what you are going through. In fact, many loved ones have a hard time understanding this illness. William Styron experienced it this way: "Depression is a disorder of mood, so mysteriously painful and elusive . . . as to verge close to being beyond description. It thus remains nearly incomprehensible to those who have not experienced it in its extreme mode." He understands the challenge that is facing you, trying to bring your loved ones on board to something that may be difficult for them to understand.

It is important to protect your own health by managing these relationships well. The question is, How do you get through these stressful encounters? The first step is to remind yourself that you have a biological illness that is treatable, and that you are doing your best to manage it. Understand the nature of your illness, its ups and downs, and your patterns. Use your treatment team wisely as a support. Then try to increase the level of understanding about the illness among your friends and family. Use assertiveness skills and effective listening techniques in your encounters with them, as outlined in chapter 9. Offer your loved ones books to read, have them come to a family meeting with your therapist, or ask them to attend a community lecture or presentation with you on mood disorders, such as those offered by NAMI (figure 10.1).

FAMILY AND FRIENDS WHO ARE SUPPORTIVE

These are the close, important people in your life, and they should be the ones you turn to during the good and not-so-good times. They should be your regular social contacts and the people you reach out to as part of your Action Plan for Relapse Prevention (for when things get worse—see chapter 7). Do not hesitate to open up to them about your illness and tell them what you are feeling, even if you are feeling suicidal. Try to have more than one person in this category, because anyone can be away or busy with life's obligations at any given moment.

FAMILY AND FRIENDS WHO ARE NOT SUPPORTIVE

Remember that not everyone is able to understand or come to terms with a mood disorder for their own reasons, which are not related to you personally.

FIGURE 10.1. **Managing relationships with family and friends**

Help your loved ones learn about your illness. Offer them books to read, or ask them to join you in a lecture or family meeting.

Use assertiveness skills and effective listening with family and friends.

Use your treatment team as a support.

Understand that you have a treatable illness with ups and downs that come in your own pattern.

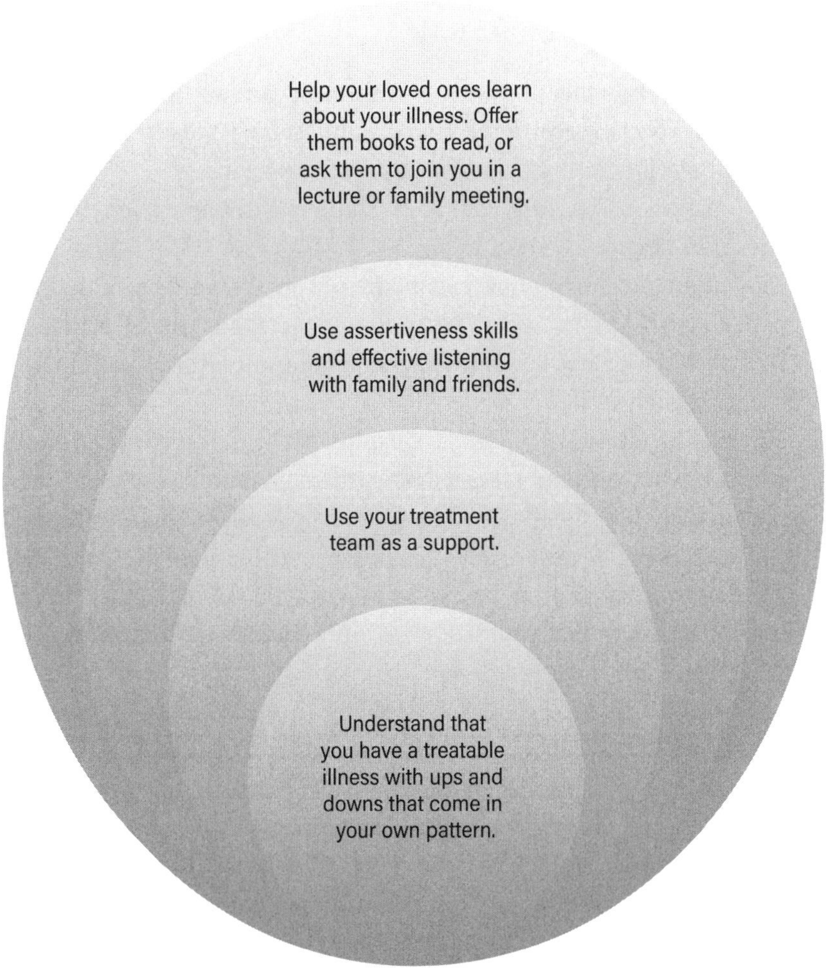

Often other people respond to your illness based on something inside themselves, not you. Some people incorrectly believe in a stigma about your illness and can see it only as shameful and socially unacceptable. They may be judgmental and critical of you, believing you to be incompetent, weak in character, or undesirable because you have a mood disorder. But this is all because of their own ill-informed belief system about mental health.

Their reactions probably feel hurtful to you, because you want your loved ones to be on your side, to fully understand your illness and what you are going through. In these situations, try to step back and understand that you may never be able to change the other person's opinion no matter how hard you try. You may need to "agree to disagree" on this matter if you want to continue the relationship. Remember that the people who respond in this way do still love you in their own way. They are just not capable of accepting your illness at this point in their lives.

- Try for a family meeting with your therapist and see if that helps.
- Do not expect to receive the kind of support from them that you might receive from other, more supportive persons.
- You may choose to limit your conversations with them to other topics, not your illness.
- You might choose to limit the amount of contact you have with this unsupportive individual, in person, on the telephone, or by text or e-mail. This is particularly important if your interactions with them are upsetting to you.
- Unfortunately, sometimes relationships, particularly new friendships, are lost when one has a mood disorder. This is painful, but again, try not to take it personally. The lost friendship is related to the other person's inability to deal with the illness, not you. You need to grieve this loss and move on as best as you can. If you shove it under the rug, saying it doesn't really matter, it will only come back to haunt you.

PEOPLE YOU CHOOSE NOT TO TELL

You have every right to keep your illness confidential and disclose it only to those closest to you. This is advisable in many situations, such as for people you have just met or recent acquaintances you do not know very well. You may also choose to keep it private from your employer and co-workers. This depends on your work situation, the type of work you do, the length of time you have worked there, your relationship with your boss, your seniority in your job, and many other factors. You may just decide to take an "extended lunch" for a doctor's appointment and say nothing more. It is all up to you—there is no right or wrong answer here.

If your illness is beginning to interfere with your job performance, however, it may then be preferable to disclose it confidentially to your employer so that he or she has a realistic understanding of why your previously outstanding work has slipped. Then together you might decide to modify your duties, change to a part-time schedule, or take some time off while you recover. You may be surprised to find out that most employers would understand.

WHEN TO DISCLOSE YOUR ILLNESS

This is a very personal decision. Choosing the right person and the right timing to reveal something about yourself and your mood disorder is difficult. Whom you disclose to, whether you do, when you do, and just how much information to give them are all very tough decisions. It depends first on your relationship with the person, the type of relationship it is (friend, family, work, or just an acquaintance), and how close you are with her. You want it to be someone you really trust and feel is supportive. Ask yourself: Is she an intimate friend or just a casual acquaintance? Do I think she will understand?

With most close and trusted family members and some close friends in your inner circle, you may want to tell them your diagnosis and reassure them that you are receiving appropriate treatment. It's best to do this only if you think they are open to hearing it and being supportive. If not, then it's not helpful to you to disclose this kind of private information no matter who the person is. Social friends, distant relatives, and casual acquaintances have no need to know. Co-workers don't need to know unless your illness affects them or their safety directly. Some examples of occupations that might require disclosure to co-workers are construction work on a scaffolding, driving a bus or train, being responsible for patient care and dispensing medications, or taking care of babies and small children.

As far as telling your boss or supervisor, you might say that you have a treatable biologically based illness that can affect your functioning and that you need some time to be treated so you can continue to do well in your job. You don't need to tell him what it is or that it is a psychiatric illness. If physical safety is an issue in your job, such as in high construction or firefighting, then you have to discuss your diagnosis with your supervisor and reassure him that both you and your co-workers are going to be safe.

HOW TO DISCLOSE YOUR ILLNESS

Go slowly and be careful about how much information you tell a person at the very beginning. Your best approach may be to speak in simple language and give them a little bit of information at a time. See how they handle receiving that, and whether they remain supportive. Gradually you can then add more detail as they can accept it. Reinforce that you have a treatable biologically based illness. If they ask questions, respond directly, if you know the answer. Direct them to read up on more information about depression or bipolar disorder on mental health websites like that of the National Alliance on Mental Illness (www.nami.org) and others that will answer some of their questions and reassure them. Remind her that this is a conversation in confidence and not to repeat it to anyone.

In speaking with your boss or supervisor, you might say that the treatment requires you to attend a certain number of appointments over the next few months. Emphasize that you're very interested in your position (or the department or company) and are committed to doing a good job. Try to get as many of your mental health appointments scheduled at the very beginning or end of the day, after work hours, or on your day off. That way, you can then go in to work an hour later or leave an hour later than usual—not generally a big problem unless you have to be home for small children. This will interfere less with your job, and your boss or co-workers won't have to cover for your absence as much.

Then do your best to stay calm while working and do a good job while there. This might require taking extra time, coming in early or late, to complete projects if you feel your concentration is lacking or your pace is slow. You might have to pay attention to workarounds, like writing yourself messages on sticky notes and keeping a calendar to remember meetings and deadlines. Know that some employers may arrange to have their employees take part-time hours or a medical leave of absence if they need extensive or prolonged treatment, and by law they are required to hold the job for them.

MANAGING RELATIONSHIPS CAN BE TRICKY

Relationships can be very tricky to handle if one or both of the persons is under stress or going through an emotional problem like depression or bipolar disorder. Sometimes the healthier spouse is not as understanding of your illness and may try to do things her own way, going as far as trying to control or manipulate you. This is not healthy for you or the relationship.

A good first step is always to sit down and have an open, honest discussion with your loved one about the problems you are having. Try to maintain a cool and composed attitude and not react with an emotional outburst, as that will only make the person defensive and escalate an argument. Your partner who has depression may not be willing to open up and share answers that only he can provide, or may offer responses that only make sense to him, not you. You might get the feeling that he is not being forthcoming or truthful in sharing all the important information with you that, in a perfect world, you would need to have. This can often cause you more distress and confusion. If you're the one who has a mood disorder, be particularly careful to listen closely and not jump to judgment too quickly. Depression can cause you to think negatively, which can affect your relationships. So stop and don't jump to conclusions without the facts.

After working hard to solve your problems, you might have to move forward in your life, with or without this person by your side. Again, trust your instincts to tell you if or when something is not right. Try to get as much solid information or evidence on which to base your decision, perhaps engaging the help of another family member or therapist who knows you well, to know when it is time to make a change. Stay away from rumors or idle gossip. When you base your decision on solid evidence, you have a better chance of making a sound decision. A person who recognizes that it is time to move forward in life has the advantage in achieving a happier outcome.

HOW TO SURVIVE THE HOLIDAYS WITH FAMILY

During the holidays many of us are surrounded by people and environments that are wrapped up in the joy and chaos of the season. If you are suffering from depression or bipolar depression, this can be a more stressful, burdensome, and irritating time than usual. When your mood and energy levels are down, it is often difficult to muster the effort to participate in holiday activities, especially since you may have no interest in doing so. That is part of the illness. But at the same time, you may feel pressure to participate, either from within or from family members.

The holiday season brings an enormous amount of stress for some, especially those with depression.

An upset in your daily routine by attending holiday-related social functions, shopping in crowded malls, or making holiday-related meals and gifts for loved ones can be more unsettling than you realize. Small changes in one's daily routine are thought to challenge the body's ability to maintain stability, and those with mood disorders may have a more difficult time adapting to these changes in routine.

Another source of stress is getting together with family members or friends you may have not seen in a long time and with whom you may feel you no longer have much in common. You may feel it as an obligation and not a joy of the season, and you may dread the anticipated unpleasant interaction but do it for the sake of "family." This is true whether one is suffering from depression or not. Families come with all sorts of members who have many different personalities and quirks. Some of them you may get along with just fine—some not so well. Some you may just have to tolerate for the sake of peace in the family. And some know just how to push your buttons! For example, your dad may always ask about your job in just that certain way that grates on you, Grandma only wants to know if you have a boyfriend or are married yet, and Uncle Eddy thinks it is funny to make jokes at your expense. You can choose to suffer them in silence, speak up and run the risk of defensive arguments with people who may never change, stay at home, or go elsewhere for the holiday.

> Stress is an emotionally and physically disturbing condition you may have in response to certain life events. During the holidays, this stress includes the change in daily routine and the overload of responsibilities common at this time of year.

Holiday stress often begins with a "should" list that is bound to get anyone into trouble. I *"should" do this or go to that function or get that gift. I "should" prepare a holiday feast for my family or make a handmade gift like Martha Stewart.* You may tend to take on an overload of responsibilities and feel guilty if you cannot live up to that self-imposed standard. Or when depressed, you may not feel like doing any of it and then feel guilty later for ignoring your loved ones. Do what you can realistically this year. Instead of saying "I should" do this or that, replace it with "I would like" to do this or that. And then, if possible, aim for your more realistic goal and don't be upset if you cannot reach it today.

Expectations are tricky. During the holidays, they often appear as an artificial set of standards that you impose on yourself, based on some unreachable ideal in a magazine, on television or the internet, or on what your great-grandmother was said to have done. Trying to reach these unrealistic expectations will only bring you disappointment and more stress, not pleasure. Instead, think about where you are with your depression, and what you can realistically do *now* for yourself and your family. Set out small goals for your holiday season, ones that are attainable. Keep it all very simple and you and others will enjoy it more.

You can manage the holidays and lessen the effect of stressful events by using coping strategies. First, maintain a regular schedule of daily activities, including diet/nutrition, sleep, daily exercise, and self-care. Enjoy the holiday food but don't overeat and be sorry later. Try to prioritize your responsibilities and activities and don't overschedule, if possible. Keep a calendar and make lists of what you have to do. Use problem-solving strategies as well as relaxation and self-soothing techniques regularly. Use humor to distract your mind—a funny book or movie often works wonders. Try mindfulness meditation, explained in chapter 9. Take a step back and learn to say no if necessary during this time so that you do not overcommit yourself.

What if you are among those who do not have a large network of family or friends to surround you? Perhaps you live in a different part of the country from your family and cannot travel, or your loved ones have passed away. Perhaps your circle of close friends has dwindled, and you are left feeling quite alone.

> Beware of the word "should." We all have a desire to please others by making the holidays picture-card perfect, but that is not reality.

The media often makes this worse, with images of groups of seemingly happy people gathering in celebration for Thanksgiving, Hanukkah, Christmas, New Year's Eve, Fourth of July, or summer vacations. When you are depressed, this visual image may seem to be everywhere you go, with little or no escape. It's often easy to forget that this is just an image and not reality, that there are many people similar to you who have just a few close connections. It's easy to forget that, in reality, people have real stressors and imperfect lives, illnesses, and financial woes and are not as "jolly" as the media image portrays. How do you get through this time of year when you *feel* so apart from those in your town?

First, ask yourself who you know well personally, and what your relationships with them are. Here is where the quality of friendship wins over quantity. Remind yourself that you are not alone in this situation, that there are many others who have a small, not large, network of family and close friends to support them. Not everyone has the life depicted in a Norman Rockwell painting or on TV. Then make an effort to connect with your network of friends. Maybe it is for a quiet lunch together, or an evening at home.

Beyond that, many people find it helpful to reach out to others in need during the holidays. Many volunteer organizations are looking for assistance, and you may find that in giving, you, too, receive something in return. Perhaps your church, synagogue, or local community center has an organization for this purpose that you can join. Try it if you are able and you may be surprised.

11

Pulling It All Together

*Managing your illness effectively means that you learn about
the illness and use certain methods, strategies, and skills
each day to respond to the symptoms you have.*

—SJN

What does it look like and feel like to manage your depression successfully, to actually do everything mentioned so far in this book? The strategies are not a magical cure for depression. But following them is a choice you make to help yourself get through the illness with episodes that are perhaps shorter and less intense.

The first thing you experience when you manage your depression is being able to go about your day with an acceptance that depression is an illness, one that can be treated and managed. It is not a weakness or a character flaw. When you manage your illness, you do not listen to those who offer misinformed comments or unhelpful advice. This is a big relief for many people. You know that as part of the illness, your mood will change up and down, and that you will have good days and not-so-good days. You try to understand the fluctuations and patterns you experience. Some days you will wake up feeling relatively okay, and other days, you will feel absolutely down. That is the time to remind yourself even more that the down times are part of the picture and that this moment will eventually pass. This is not easy to do.

When you manage your depression well, you follow the basics of mental health each day. These will help you stay well mentally and physically. Managing your depression means you keep up with personal self-care and follow the treatment plan set up with your providers. You sleep 7 to 8 hours every night, eat a balanced diet of healthy real food three times a day, limit caffeine and tobacco intake, and do not use alcohol or street drugs. It means that you take all your medications as prescribed, even if you are feeling better. It includes getting some form of exercise each day, depending on your physical limits.

Another essential piece of managing your depression well is to avoid isolation. You do this by keeping up with your family and friends and other social contacts, even when you don't really feel like it. If you have not heard from someone in a while, you pick up the phone and call the person. Sometimes other people do not know what to say to you when you feel very depressed, so they may not call for fear of feeling awkward or uncomfortable. At those times, it is important for you to initiate the contact, to keep up those friendships that will sustain you.

Following the basics of mental health means that you structure your day and follow a routine. You get up and dressed at the same time each day and have several things planned, written down in a calendar or agenda book, paper or electronic. You pace yourself with a realistic number of activities that you can accomplish. These include your responsibilities and obligations, pleasurable and positive experiences, and mastery experiences (see chapter 8). You understand that it is not helpful for you to stay in bed or on the couch all day, with endless hours of free time on your hands. You know how difficult it is to go to work or be active when you are depressed and tired and don't have an interest in anything. The best advice is to do it anyway, and motivation will eventually follow. Many people have found that they start off feeling too tired to do something, but when they become engaged in the project, the fatigue seems to get better or disappear.

Managing your depression effectively requires that you pay attention to your symptoms and monitor them. You are aware of your specific warning signs and triggers for worsening depression. You have made a plan with your treatment team to intervene when a change in these signs becomes problematic. In that plan, you know what measures to take and whom to contact for help. Managing your illness well also means that you take steps to minimize the chance of relapse occurring and to keep yourself safe. You do this by following the basic preventive steps summarized above, which will help you maintain emotional stability and decrease your vulnerability to fluctuations. You learn to use effective coping skills in the short and long term to help get you through the rough patches. This means that you identify in advance what is pleasurable, relaxing, and distracting for you and are ready to engage in those activities when needed. You use problem-solving techniques and avoid negative behaviors. You learn to navigate the pathways of families and intimate relationships and recruit the greatest support possible.

All of the above prepares you to do the really hard work of managing depression, which is learning how to control the negative, distorted thoughts and self-talk that seem to dominate your mind and upset you. This is not easy to do, and it may take years to develop the skill. You learn to identify a negative thought when it appears and understand that it is the depression talking, that it is not a fact. You learn to challenge the negative thought and replace it with a more realistic one. When you understand the source of the negative thought, you take away the power it has over your thinking and in turn your mood.

You may wonder how you can follow these recommendations to manage your illness when you are depressed and feel no hope. It is helpful for you to believe in the exercises to get the most benefit from them, but not essential. Do them anyway. If you do not feel hopeful about your future, *borrow some hope* from a person you respect, someone who knows and understands you. Tell yourself, "Jon believes there is hope for me, and he is no fool." Eventually you will find that the hope is your own.

None of this comes easily, but with continued effort and practice, you will be able to manage your depression and increase your chance of staying well.

Collective Wisdom

Beware of false knowledge; it is more dangerous than ignorance.
—GEORGE BERNARD SHAW

ADVICE FROM SOME REMARKABLE PEOPLE

Do not buy into these [negative, distorted] thoughts.
Not fair to believe them. Wait it out.
—TIMOTHY J. PETERSEN

A very wise clinical psychologist reminded me of this one day when I was feeling particularly low and hopeless about my situation, overwhelmed with negative thoughts, which he believed were untrue and distorted. My depressed brain believed these thoughts were true and would last forever, a common belief in depression. It was easier to believe these thoughts than to do the work of challenging them, particularly when so depressed.

His point was that these thoughts were the depression talking, and that they would not last forever. He said that it was not fair to me to believe something that was not true, something that was based on the disease, even though my brain was trying to tell me otherwise. He asked me to be patient and wait until the negative, distorted thoughts passed. This was not easy to do, but with our work together and time, they eventually did. I try to remind myself of this each time the negative thoughts become intrusive.

The time you are feeling the worst is not the time to give up!
—ANDREW A. NIERENBERG

Again, this advice came from an extraordinarily wise and clever psychiatrist at a dark and hopeless time in my life. I was ready to call it quits, and he was just *not* going to let that happen. He wrote this statement on a paper prescription pad and signed it. I still keep the paper in my wallet. His point was that we should not make major life decisions, such as giving up, when we are very down and depressed, at our lowest point. When you are feeling the worst, you are not in a position to make the best decisions for yourself and may do something that you will later regret. At the time, you don't realize it and may think that you are capable of making a reasonable decision—your depressed brain is telling you to go ahead with it. His plea was to wait until I was feeling better to make any major life decisions. He was clever, because of course, when I felt better, I did not want to give up! So, in this way, he got me to keep going and not give up.

> *Feelings are not fact. Interpretation is not fact. Judgment is not fact. STOP. Look at the facts. Then modify your assessment/interpretation of the situation.*
> —TIMOTHY J. PETERSEN

This was a reminder from my therapist when I struggled with believing my distorted thoughts were facts. He reminded me that in depression, negative events are magnified and may dominate your thinking. When you are depressed, you are more likely to believe that biased or distorted thoughts are true. Remember: thoughts and feelings are not facts. Feelings are created by your thoughts and your interpretations of an event, not by the actual event. Do not confuse feelings and thoughts with facts. Stop and look at the situation in front of you, at the objective facts of the situation. Then make your own assessment based on these facts and not based on any distorted thoughts or feelings. Doing this will bring you to a more realistic view of the situation and cause you less distress.

> *With depression, feeling "good" is alien and may feel uncomfortable at first. You are not used to it and may feel anxious. The brain sees it as different and "not right," so the tendency is to go back. Don't. You have to push yourself.*
> —M. JACOBO

Here, a therapist was preparing me for the idea of making progress in therapy. The statement points out that when you are immersed in a mental state like depression for a long time, the brain gets used to it and sees any change from depression as "different." So, when you start to feel good, that new "feel good" state may feel "bad" or uncomfortable to you. You might feel anxious, irritable, and out of sorts. You might feel like retreating back to your old depressed self, which is familiar. Do not allow that to happen. You have to push yourself to get used to the new idea of feeling "good," or at least "better," and eventually you will adjust to it. After all, that is your ultimate goal.

> *Practice consciously endorsing yourself.*
> —M. JACOBO

Most people who suffer from depression are very good at negative self-talk. Finding negative, critical things to say about themselves seems to come easily. "I am a loser" and "I am no good" are fairly universal (and inaccurate) beliefs among those who have this illness. But this is not healthy for you. With depression, you have to learn to think about yourself in more positive terms and to give yourself credit for your accomplishments, no matter how small. You have to practice endorsing yourself, on purpose, consciously, and get comfortable having those positive thoughts in your head. Practice saying "I am a good _____" (fill in the blank) several times a day until it feels natural to you. That is what my therapist was trying to say in this statement.

> *Action precedes motivation.*
> —MCLEAN HOSPITAL MAP PROGRAM (original source Robert J. McKain)

This is said so often, it has become the mantra of the McLean Hospital Partial Hospital Mood and Anxiety Program. It is meant to address the inertia that comes with depression, the lack of interest in life and in doing things (called anhedonia). What it means is that even when you are depressed and don't feel like doing anything, you should go ahead and do something anyway. Do not wait until you feel like doing it, because in depression, that will not come for a very long time. If you begin to do things, eventually the motivation to do them will follow. It is far easier to stay in bed or on the couch, but that is not in your best interest. Just get going on some small thing and eventually the interest in doing it will follow, and you will become interested in more things. Start with one small thing at a time, and the motivation for doing it will later appear.

> *Sometimes we experience a combination of physical, emotional, and interpersonal symptoms for such a long time that we don't even recognize them as symptoms. We get used to them and think they are normal.*
> —MARJORIE HANSEN SHAEVITZ

We discussed this in group therapy years ago, and I just now discovered who wrote it, although it is taken from a book I have not read. I know that it is very true in depression. When symptoms persist for a long time, and your memory gets fuzzy, it is hard to remember what your past self was like. When you get used to the symptoms of long-standing depression, you may think of it as your "normal" self. Remember—that is not true. It is not your normal self. The exercise in chapter 4 is designed to help you define your baseline healthy self and have that as a goal to work toward during your recovery.

> *Courage doesn't always roar. Sometimes courage is the quiet voice*
> *at the end of the day saying, "I will try again tomorrow."*
> —MARY ANNE RADMACHER

This quotation speaks volumes to me. Depression is the kind of illness that requires a lot of courage. Many of us go around with this illness in silence, not mentioning it to any but a few of our closest friends and family, quietly struggling. It takes a lot of effort just to get up each day, to get showered and dressed and try. It takes enormous courage to get up and face another day of depression, of darkness and despair and hopelessness. When you are willing to do that day after day, you have courage unlike any other. You do not have to shout it from the rooftops—you show it quietly by your efforts.

> *You cannot absorb praise unless you decide to*
> *believe and validate what is being said.*
> —MGH PSYCHIATRY RESIDENT

A psychiatry resident said this to me one day during one of my major struggles. It is meaningful to those with depression who are overwhelmed with negative self-talk and beliefs that interfere with their ability to receive praise or a compliment. She meant to say that you need to be able to respect and believe what the other person is saying, and validate them, before you can absorb the positive comments they are offering you. That is not easy to do. Once you decide that you can trust and believe the other person, then you can accept their words as accurate and complimentary.

> *There is Hope because . . . we see you in a different way than*
> *you see yourself, and if you were to see yourself as we see you,*
> *then you could believe and hope that life could be different.*
> —JONATHAN E. ALPERT

I was struggling terribly with the idea of having no hope for a life when this wise psychiatrist said this to me. I had to learn and later accept that he saw me in a different way than I saw myself. I was looking through depressed glasses and could not see things as he did, a common problem in depression. And since he saw me differently, he saw a potential for life and hope that I was unable to envision when depressed. I am still learning to see myself through his eyes and the eyes of others who see me this way, to see my potential through their point of view.

> *That is just the way you have come to regard yourself.*
> *It is not necessarily true.*
> —APS PHYSICIAN

Another physician, who did not know me at all, picked up on the extremely negative view of myself that in depression my brain had come to believe as true. In one brief encounter, she understood that my self-view was an inaccurate distortion. It blew the roof off my long-held premise that the whole world knew me to be as I saw myself when she challenged it. It became a turning point for me, to have someone quickly see through to the "old" me, who was not as my depressed self envisioned. I have to constantly remind myself of her words that this is "not necessarily true."

> *We cannot direct the winds, but we can adjust our sails.*
> —THOMAS S. MONSON

I found this quotation on a coaster! It has many applications to our lives whether we are depressed or not. The underlying message is that many things happen in our lives that we cannot avoid or control. We could do nothing and become victims. Our best approach is to be flexible and adapt to what we are unable to control. The "winds" here represent outside influences, other people, mother nature, and just what life throws at you. Sometimes it's a loss of a loved one, a job or a relationship, an illness, or when things don't happen to go your way. These all can have a powerful influence on us. We can't usually do anything to modify these challenges in life, other than adapt and change our approach. Adjusting your sails might mean that you make choices that take you down a slightly different path than you had imagined for yourself, or put some things on hold for a while. At times the storms are powerful; we feel beat up and our sails become torn. We might need added perseverance and resilience just to stay afloat. This quotation reminds us that we need to be flexible in life, constantly adjusting ourselves and our path in response to the world.

> *The greatest weapon against stress is our ability to choose*
> *one thought [or action] over another.*
> —WILLIAM JAMES

William James is a well-known American psychologist and philosopher from the twentieth century. I like this quotation because it speaks to the fact that we all have a choice, and what we choose to think or do has an effect on our lives, on our ability to manage stress and other challenges. I believe this includes our ability to deal with a mood disorder, as we can see that changing a negative thought or behavior with CBT exercises can change the course of an episode of depression.

> *Beware of false knowledge; it is more dangerous than ignorance.*
> —GEORGE BERNARD SHAW

An Irish author and playwright, Shaw reminds us here to use reliable resources in our quest for information, and beware of the partial, inaccurate, and skewed viewpoints circulating around us. It translates to this decade, as we now have a wide variety of sites on the internet that don't always have solid evidence to back up their statements. (See tables 12.1 and 12.2 for tips on evaluating information online.) He reminds us that random sources can create potential harm if believed and followed, more so than having no knowledge of the issue. When that extends to your health, including mental health, it may lead to a delay in diagnosis and treatment, unnecessary suffering from an improperly treated illness, or worsening of your condition.

> *The best kind of people . . . make you see the sun where you once saw clouds.*
> *The people that believe in you so much, you start to believe in you too.*
> —KATE LATTEY, *AGAINST THE CLOCK*

My friend Ginger is a great example of this. She proves to me that having good support from your inner circle of friends can change the way you think about yourself and the world. Their input can affect the outlook you have on your day or week. More important, the best relationships can improve your self-esteem, self-confidence, and belief in yourself when you begin to see yourself as others see you. Good people, whom you respect, would not be supportive of you if you had no redeemable qualities, if you truly were a "loser"! The lesson here is, choose your friends wisely, reserving your closest relationships for those who will be supportive during your ups and downs.

Health is a state of complete physical, mental and social well-being,
and not merely the absence of disease or infirmity.
—WORLD HEALTH ORGANIZATION

This is a new way of thinking about health and wellness compared to the thinking just a generation ago. It moves away from a focus solely on the physical to thinking about the whole person in context. This principle is important because it emphasizes that health is more than just the absence of symptoms; the definition extends to all aspects of a person's being.

I guess in the end . . . what matters is what
we chose to do with the things we had.
—MIRA GRANT

I love this quotation! First, it reminds us that we all have choices in life. Second, it reminds us that everyone has been given a different set of skills, abilities, resources, opportunities, and tools to get through life. Few of us have it perfect. The important thing is what you do with what you have to work with. Some of us will persevere and strive toward a goal. Some may also be more resilient to adversity if or when that occurs. Unfortunately, others may be content to just sit back, passively allowing things to happen "to" them, not advocating for themselves or meeting life's challenges. It's like the old cliché in a card game—you have to do the best with the hand (cards) you are dealt.

TECHNOLOGY IN MENTAL ILLNESS

In recent years several computer-based monitoring, psychoeducation, and therapy programs for depression, bipolar disorder, anxiety, stress, substance abuse, and eating disorders have emerged. They have shown some effectiveness as well as some challenges. Mobile phones may be suited to mental health care delivery in some instances, particularly as they are portable and are the preferred method of communication among young people, an age group commonly affected by mood disorders and sometimes reluctant to seek treatment. Self-monitoring on a mobile phone app is easy to use and may allow for increased adherence to treatment with real-time monitoring, reminder prompts, and delivery of simple self-management strategies, information, and tips.

It's important to be aware of a few things before choosing online therapy. First, it lacks the interpersonal interaction and chemistry between therapist and client that has made therapy so effective. Psychotherapy works in part because therapists offer a safe, confidential space to share deeply private and personal stories, thoughts, and emotions with real-time feedback. Electronic therapy apps are still a new technology and may not be the right tool for everyone. They lack the interpersonal qualities and feedback so essential to the success of talk therapy, yet they might be of use if you live in a remote geographic area and cannot easily get in to meet with a therapist.

If you try online therapy, be sure to find out if the therapists are licensed in their state and in your state. Ask if the site or app is secure, and if the information you provide is confidential. Will you have to pay for the service, and will your insurance plan cover it? Online sites may be helpful in conjunction with office-based person-to-person treatment and as a way to send text messages or track and log moods or thoughts.

Helpful Mobile Apps

Some *mental health apps* available on smartphones and other mobile devices are relevant to depression, anxiety, insomnia, and other mental health conditions. There are also apps for your exercise and nutrition needs, which I discuss in chapter 1. It's hard to know which apps are the most helpful to your specific interests and needs. I recommend checking out PsyberGuide (www.psyberguide.org), a nonprofit website for consumers dedicated to the review and rating of mental health apps for mental health conditions, including mood disorders, and related treatments, such as cognitive behavioral therapy. You'll find what you need there. The internet also has social media sites with blogs and chat rooms related to depression. DBSA (Depression and Bipolar Support Alliance), the International Bipolar Foundation, and Psychology Today online are good places to start, as well as the Mood Network, discussed below.

Research Studies Using Technology

One research group recently looked at the effect of smartphone-based mental health interventions for depression. They combined the results (data) from eighteen eligible randomized controlled trials (RCTs) who used twenty-two smartphone apps in 3,414 participants. The way they combined the results is called a *meta-analysis*, a tool in statistics that researchers use to analyze the combined results from multiple research studies, looking at the combined treatment effect. When the treatment effect is consistent across these multiple studies, it gives us meaningful information.

This meta-analysis showed that the use of these twenty-two smartphone mental health interventions had a moderately positive effect on reducing depressive symptoms compared to a control group. Smartphone interventions based on CBT, mindfulness training, and mood monitoring significantly reduced depressive symptoms. The researchers' conclusion in reviewing these eighteen studies is that smartphone apps can effectively be used as a self-management tool for those who have less severe levels of depression. Future studies are needed.

Another research study, called the BRIGHTEN study, conducted by Patricia Areán at the University of Washington, is remarkable in that it used a smartphone app to deliver treatment interventions for depression and actually conduct the RCT. Data are still being analyzed, but early results show that it had a significant effect on mood and disability over time (www.nimh.nih.gov/news/science-news/2016/a-bright-technological-future-for-mental-health-trials.shtml).

A group in Australia described the use of a mobile app called myCompass, an interactive self-help program that includes real-time self-monitoring with message prompts and brief cognitive behavioral therapy modules. Users can track their moods, symptoms, and behaviors, schedule reminders, receive graphical feedback, and learn about mental health conditions, helpful tips, and strategies. It is designed for those who have mild to moderate depression, anxiety, and stress. Preliminary analysis showed a reduction in symptoms and overall psychological distress after using myCompass. The researchers support the use of mobile interventions with the potential of improving psychological well-being.

Researchers in Denmark have planned a project using smartphone-based monitoring and treatment to reduce the rate and duration of readmission among those who have unipolar depression and bipolar disorder. Called the RADMIS project, it will also help to provide clinical evidence for improving depression symptoms in those who have a mood disorder (www.cachet.dk/news/2016/03/ifd-radmis).

Another series of three studies looked at the use of a brief gamelike mobile app used on any device that connects to the internet. The app, called Therapeutic Evaluative Conditioning (TEC), is designed to increase aversion to self-injurious thoughts and behaviors, like self-cutting and suicidal plans and behaviors. It was shown to decrease most of these behaviors except suicidal thoughts. Future studies are needed.

The Mood Network is a confidential online research project that provides a way for individuals who have depression or bipolar disorder to advance scientific knowledge about their condition while also receiving helpful information and support. It's a brand new approach to doing research in psychiatry, an online collaboration between those who have depression or bipolar disorder, clinicians, and researchers in psychiatry. The Mood Network is a partnership that respects the person who has depression as an "expert-by-experience" in the effort to find which treatment, therapies, and practice work best for which type of symptoms and which person. The Mood Network's goal is to engage 50,000 people with depression or bipolar disorder in their online studies. Information gained from the studies, which is confidential, will contribute to a pool of data that will now be large enough for researchers to figure out which treatments work best for which kind of mood disorders in which people.

Here's how it works. The Mood Network is based online at https://mood network.org. It's free. It's confidential. To participate, you create your own username and password to log on to the Mood Network website. Then you are able to access the Mood Network's blogs and forums (discussion groups), where you are free to read about other people's opinions and experiences with their illness, side effects, different treatments, and so on. You can also confidentially post your own comments or respond to what others have written. The Mood Network researchers pay great attention to what is posted in these sections.

There is also a place where you can ask questions of an expert clinician and give your feedback on what is important to you in terms of areas of research for them to focus on. You can go to a section called "How am I doing?" and take a questionnaire or two to see if you currently have depression or mania, and then track your progress through time.

In addition, the Mood Network has continuing online research studies that you can choose to participate in, confidentially, such as the benefits of doing yoga with a certain online video or the use of a particular smartphone application in mood disorders. The Mood Network uses all this information, confidentially, to understand how people are doing in general and what treatments they have found to be helpful. They link that info about helpful treatments (confidentially) to the type of symptoms, which we know varies among people.

For additional websites with useful information for people who have mood disorders, see table 12.3.

TABLE 12.1. Evaluating Health Information on the Internet

THINGS TO CONSIDER	WHY IS THIS IMPORTANT?
Why do I need to evaluate information on the internet?	You need to be able to find reliable health-related information from trustworthy sources and avoid false or misleading health claims that can be found on the internet. This means that you must know the sources of the information.
Who runs the website?	You need to know who is responsible for a website and its content to be able to evaluate the accuracy and reliability of the information. Look for an "About Us" page and the site's editorial board.
Who pays for it?	An organization that sponsors, or pays for, a website can influence the type and amount of information provided and how it is presented. To evaluate health information, you must first identify any possible *slant* or *bias* in the material presented. For example, the accuracy of health-related information presented may be influenced by a company's desire to sell a product or service.
What is its *purpose?*	This is related to who sponsors it. A website's goal could be patient education, fundraising, or business. This can present a possible slant or bias. It is important to understand a website's purpose when evaluating the information presented.
Where does the information come from?	To evaluate the quality and reliability of health information, you need to understand where it comes from. The website should identify the following: • The original source of the information—who wrote it. The source should be a person or organization known to have knowledge and expertise in the area. The site should identify material written by the website staff. • The scientific evidence on which the health information is based, including references for medical facts and statistics (numbers).

(*continued*)

TABLE 12.1. **Evaluating Health Information on the Internet**

THINGS TO CONSIDER	WHY IS THIS IMPORTANT?
Where does the information come from? (*continued*)	• Individual opinions as "opinion" and clearly separated from medical information that is based on sound research *(evidence-based information)*. • The medical credentials of the author(s) and reviewers to demonstrate that they have expertise in the topic (professional degrees, training, positions).
When was it written?	The information presented should be recent and up-to-date. It should be reviewed regularly to provide you with current information. The most recent *update* or *review date* should be posted on the website.
What different types of health-related material can be found on websites?	• *Statements* or facts supported by scientific evidence and research • *Statements* not supported by scientific evidence • *Opinions* by recognized experts on the topic (editorials, comments) • *Opinions* by someone who is not a recognized expert on the topic • *Personal stories* (case reports) • A *combination* of science-based fact and clinical experience by recognized experts in the field
Is the information *reviewed* by experts?	Health-related websites should state whether their information is reviewed before posting, by whom, and ideally how this is done. The process usually involves: • a review of the scientific articles *(evidence)* from respected medical journals • an evaluation of how and why the information is important *(relevance)* • a concise summary of the important points • identification of the authors and their credentials • a review of the material by other medical professionals with expertise in the topic *(peer reviewed)*

THINGS TO CONSIDER	WHY IS THIS IMPORTANT?
How reliable are the *links* to other sites?	Websites can choose to include links to other websites. Their policy could be based on whether other sites meet certain standards or criteria, or they might include only those outside websites that pay them for advertising or to be included.
What about my *privacy?*	Websites track what pages in the site you are viewing. They may use this information to improve or modify their site. You may be asked to "register" with the website, sometimes for a fee. When you register, you give some *personal information* to the website. The site should explain what it does with your personal information. You should understand the website's privacy policy. Some sites may sell your information to other companies. Do not register for anything that makes you uncomfortable.
Are users able to *communicate* with the website?	Websites should offer a way for users (like you) to contact them with questions, problems, and feedback. If there is a chat room or online discussion area, the site should disclose the terms of service, how it is monitored, and by whom.

Source: Adapted in part from US Department of Health and Human Services, "How to Evaluate Health Information on the Internet," accessed January 2018, https://ods.od.nih.gov/Health_Information/How _To_Evaluate_Health_Information_on_the_Internet_Questions_and_Answers.aspx.

TABLE 12.2. **Classifying Web Addresses: Clues in the Name**

WEB ADDRESS ENDING IN	TYPE OF ORGANIZATION THAT RUNS IT	EXAMPLES
.gov	Federal government-sponsored sites	• National Institutes of Health
.edu	Schools and other educational institutions	• A medical school • A university
.org	Noncommercial organizations	• American Psychiatric Association • A hospital
.com	Commercial organizations (businesses)	• A drug company • A bookstore

HELPFUL WEBSITES

TABLE 12.3. **Helpful Websites**

U.S. GOVERNMENT RESOURCES

- National Institute of Mental Health
  Information about depression and bipolar disorder, including current research and clinical trials
  www.nimh.nih.gov

MENTAL HEALTH ORGANIZATIONS

- American Psychiatric Association
  Patient educational information about depression and bipolar disorder
  www.psych.org
  www.psychiatry.org/depression
  www.psychiatry.org/bipolar

- American Psychological Association
  Patient educational information about depression and bipolar disorder
  www.apa.org

- Depression and Bipolar Support Alliance (National Manic Depressive and Depressive Association)
  An educational resource for patients with depression, with information on support groups and educational programs
  www.dbsalliance.org

- National Alliance on Mental Illness
  Information about depression and other mental illness
  www.nami.org

- International Bipolar Foundation
  A nonprofit organization dedicated to improving understanding and treatment of bipolar disorder through research; promoting care and support services for individuals and caregivers; and erasing stigma through education
  www.ibpf.org

SUPPORT GROUPS

- PatientsLikeMe
  A website where you can compare your symptoms and progress in real time with others who share your diagnosis
  www.patientslikeme.com

(continued)

TABLE 12.3. **Helpful Websites**

SUPPORT GROUPS (continued)

- BeyondBlue
  An independent nonprofit organization supported by the federal government of Australia, with information for patients with depression and bipolar disorder.

www.beyondblue.org.au

SLEEP RESOURCES

- American Academy of Sleep Medicine
  Professional association website with some links to patient educational sites

www.aasmnet.org
www.sleepeducation.org

- US National Institutes of Health / National Heart, Lung, and Blood Institute
  Your Guide to Healthy Sleep

www.nhlbi.nih.gov/files/docs
/public/sleep/healthy_sleep.pdf

EXERCISE RESOURCES

- Centers for Disease Control
  Physical Activity Guidelines

www.cdc.gov/physicalactivity
/basics/index.htm

- US Department of Health and Human Services
  2008 Physical Activity Guidelines for Americans

www.health.gov/PAGuidelines
/guidelines

- American College of Sports Medicine
  Exercise guidelines (found online under Public Information: Position Stands)

www.acsm.org

NUTRITION RESOURCES

- US Department of Agriculture Nutrition and Physical Activity Guidelines
  SuperTracker: an online tool to track your daily exercise and calories

www.choosemyplate.gov
/tools-supertracker

- US Department of Health and Human Services
  USDA Dietary Guidelines for Americans, 2015–2020

www.health.gov/dietaryguidelines
/2015/guidelines
www.choosemyplate.gov

- US Center for Disease Control
  Nutrition

www.cdc.gov/nutrition

BOOKS OF INTEREST

Aleem, Ashley, Jennifer Bahr, Colin Depp, et al. *Healthy Living with Bipolar Disorder*. San Diego, CA: International Bipolar Foundation, 2017.

Beck, Aaron T., A. John Rush, Brian F. Shaw, and Gary Emery. *Cognitive Therapy of Depression*. New York: Guilford Press, 1979.

Burns, David. *Feeling Good: The New Mood Therapy*. New York: Avon Books, 1980.

Copeland, Mary Ellen. *The Depression Workbook: A Guide for Living with Depression and Manic Depression*. Oakland, CA: New Harbinger, 2001.

Copeland, Mary Ellen. *Living without Depression and Manic Depression: A Workbook for Maintaining Mood Stability*. Oakland, CA: New Harbinger, 1994.

Fung, Teresa. *Healthy Eating: A Guide to the New Nutrition*. A Harvard Medical School Special Health Report. Boston: Harvard Health Publications, 2016.

Jacobs, Gregg D. *Say Goodnight to Insomnia*. New York: Owl Books, 1998.

MacKinnon, Dean F. *Still Down: What to Do When Antidepressants Fail*. Baltimore: Johns Hopkins University Press, 2016.

Mindfulness: The New Science of Health and Happiness. New York: Time Special Edition, 2017.

Newman, Cory F., Robert L. Leahy, Aaron T. Beck, and Noreen A. Reilly-Harrington. *Bipolar Disorder: A Cognitive Therapy Approach*. Washington, DC: American Psychological Association, 2002.

Noonan, Susan J. *When Someone You Know Has Depression: Words to Say and Things to Do*. Baltimore: Johns Hopkins University Press, 2016.

Sichel, Deborah, and Jeanne W. Driscoll. *Women's Moods: What Every Woman Must Know about Hormones, the Brain, and Emotional Health*. New York: Quill, 1999.

Sylvia, Louisa Grandin. *The Wellness Workbook for Bipolar Disorder: Your Guide to Getting Healthy and Improving Your Mood*. Oakland, CA: New Harbinger, 2015.

Young, Jeffrey E., and Janet S. Klosko. *Reinventing Your Life*. New York: Penguin, 1994.

Memoirs

Casey, Nell. *Unholy Ghost: Writers on Depression*. New York: William Morrow, 2001.

Ferris, Amy, ed. *Shades of Blue: Writers on Depression, Suicide and Feeling Blue*. Berkeley, CA: Seal Press, 2015.

Jamison, Kay Redfield. *Night Falls Fast: Understanding Suicide*. New York: Vintage Books, 2000.

Jamison, Kay Redfield. *Touched with Fire: Manic Depressive Illness and the Artistic Temperament*. New York: Free Press, 1993.

Jamison, Kay Redfield. *An Unquiet Mind: A Memoir of Mood and Madness*. New York: Vintage Books, 1995.

Manning, Martha. *Undercurrents: A Life beneath the Surface*. New York: HarperOne, 1995.

Styron, William. *Darkness Visible: A Memoir of Madness*. New York: Vintage Books, 1990.

Thompson, Tracy. *The Beast: A Journey through Depression*. New York: Plume, 1996.

Meditation

Benson, Herbert. *Beyond the Relaxation Response*. New York: Berkley Books, 1984.

Benson, Herbert. *The Relaxation Response*. Rev. ed. New York: Harper, 2000.

Kabat-Zinn, Jon. *Wherever You Go, There You Are*. New York: Hyperion, 1994.

Communication Skills

Booher, Dianna. *Communicate with Confidence: How to Say It Right the First Time*. New York: McGraw-Hill, 1994.

Davidson, Jeff. *The Complete Idiot's Guide to Assertiveness*. New York: Alpha Books, 1997.

Fine, Debra. *The Fine Art of Small Talk*. New York: Hyperion, 2005.

Yeung, A., G. Feldman, and M. Fava. *Self-Management of Depression: A Manual for Mental Health and Primary Care Professionals*. New York: Cambridge University Press, 2010, app. C.

Conclusion

I guess in the end ... what matters is what we
chose to do with the things we had.
—MIRA GRANT

I present a lot of material on managing your mood disorder in the chapters of this book. Starting with the basics of mental health as a foundation for staying healthy and building new skills, I then cover how to identify and monitor your mood disorder and its symptoms. Common obstacles to your recovery from a mood disorder are outlined in chapter 3. In chapter 4, I describe how to identify your baseline healthy self, why it is important, and how it will provide you with a goal for your recovery. Chapter 5 presents you with treatment options and many ways to manage your mood disorder, such as understanding your fluctuations, identifying and monitoring your warning signs and triggers, and maintaining a routine and structure. Identifying your goal in treatment, with an overview of wellness, follows in chapter 6. In chapter 7, I detail how to respond to your symptoms as they arise by developing an Action Plan and following relapse prevention strategies.

Chapter 8 describes cognitive behavioral therapy, a type of talk therapy particularly useful in depression, with several practical exercises to reinforce the principles of CBT. These CBT exercises help you challenge negative thoughts and avoid negative behaviors, both of which are common in depression. Several strategies are reviewed in chapter 9 to help you get through the difficult times: coping and stress, mindfulness, distress tolerance, communication skills, talking with your doctor, and tips for family and friends. Chapter 10 covers thoughts on dealing with friends and families, including a section on relationships and the holidays. In chapter 11, I give you a picture of what life can be like when you follow the recommendations outlined in this book. The last chapter presents additional resources, such as useful books, technology in mental health, and guidelines for using the internet to obtain health information.

Do not expect that you will master this material all in one reading. It will take time and practice to learn and incorporate these approaches into your day. Managing your mood disorder means that you learn about the illness and develop strategies to respond to your symptoms. It means that each day you use methods, strategies, and skills described in this book to deal with the symptoms you have. Managing your illness requires that you monitor your symptoms, challenge negative thoughts, use problem-solving techniques, make adjustments, and avoid negative behaviors. This is a lot to do; in fact, it may feel overwhelming to you right now. With time and practice, however, all steps outlined in this book are possible to accomplish. More important, they will make a difference in how you feel. Work with your treatment providers on this.

Do not be surprised if you need to review sections of the book periodically. Review and practice is how we all learn new skills. This book was designed to introduce the topics relevant to depression one at a time, then to help you reinforce the material by using specific exercises and examples relevant to your life. Last, this book is a reference for reviewing the material later as needed. When you come upon a section that hits home, that is particularly familiar to your situation, sit with it and think about it for a while. Consider how it relates to you. That would be a good example of something for you to discuss with your therapist or physician.

Keep in mind that people who participate actively in their care have a better chance of recovery and staying well. So keep working at it. It may take a while for you to notice a change in your mood, and this may understandably affect your motivation to follow the recommendations outlined in the book. Doing so may feel like a struggle. Just remember that action precedes motivation: take that step whether you feel like it today or not.

Good luck!

Appendix

Some Medications Used Alone or in Combination for Depression, Bipolar Disorder, Anxiety, and Sleep (brand name is in parentheses)

Selective serotonin reuptake inhibitors, SSRIs
citalopram (Celexa)
escitalopram (Lexapro)
fluoxetine (Prozac)
fluvoxamine (Luvox)
paroxetine (Paxil)
sertraline (Zoloft)

Serotonin-norepinephrine reuptake inhibitors, SNRIs
desvenlafaxine (Pristiq)
duloxetine (Cymbalta)
venlafaxine (Effexor)

Other antidepressants
bupropion (Wellbutrin)
mirtazapine (Remeron)

Tricyclic antidepressants
amitriptyline (Elavil)
clomipramine (Anafranil)
imipramine (Tofranil)
nortriptyline (Pamelor)

Monoamine oxidase inhibitors (MAOIs)
phenelzine (Nardil)
tranylcypromine (Parnate)

Mood stabilizers for bipolar disorder
carbamazepine (Tegretol)
lamotrigine (Lamictal)
lithium carbonate (Eskalith)
valproate (Depakote)

Atypical antipsychotics
aripiprazole (Abilify)
brexpiprazole (Rexulti)
clozapine (Clozaril)
lurasidone (Latuda)
olanzapine (Zyprexa)
quetiapine (Seroquel)
risperidone (Risperdal)
ziprasidone (Geodon)

Antianxiety
alprazolam (Xanax)
buspirone (Buspar)
clonazepam (Klonopin)
lorazepam (Ativan)

Alternative treatments, nonprescription, over-the-counter
Folic acid
N-acetyl cysteine
Omega-3 fatty acids
S-adenosyl-L-methionine (SAMe)

Medications used for sleep
eszopiclone (Lunesta)
melatonin
ramelteon (Rozerem)
temazepam (Restoril)
trazodone
zaleplon (Sonata)
zolpidem (Ambien)

Glossary

Action Plan for Relapse Prevention An intervention Action Plan for Relapse Prevention is a written self-care plan to help you deal with a worsening or recurrence of depression. It is a strategy you create with your doctor. You fill it out in advance and have it ready for the times when your depression symptoms start getting worse. The Action Plan helps you to identify your triggers and warning signs. It outlines the steps you will take to manage, cope, and distract from the high intensity of a depressive or manic episode. The Action Plan also lists the people you will ask to help you during these times: health care providers, family, and friends.

automatic negative thoughts In depression, the mind quickly jumps to negative thoughts, which usually cause distress. These are the thoughts that are biased in an extremely negative direction, such as "I'm a loser" or "I can't do anything right." This happens because (1) in depression, negative events dominate your thinking, and (2) the depressed mind tends to interpret and distort or twist things negatively, thus creating the negative thoughts. These thoughts happen automatically, not on purpose. Automatic negative thoughts are not an accurate reflection of reality. They are a distortion.

bipolar disorder Bipolar disorder, or manic-depressive disorder, is a relapsing and remitting, treatable mood disorder that has a major effect on daily life. Relapsing and remitting means that the episodes come and go. As with major depression, it is thought to be caused by a dysfunction in the network of neurons (brain cells) in the brain. Bipolar disorder is characterized by periodic episodes of extremely elevated mood or irritability alternating with periodic episodes of depression.

cognitive behavioral therapy Cognitive behavioral therapy (CBT) is a kind of talk therapy (psychotherapy) that addresses the connection between your thoughts, feelings, and actions. In CBT you learn to identify and change thinking patterns that may be distorted, beliefs that are inaccurate, and behaviors that are unhelpful.

cognitive distortions Distortions in your thoughts are errors in thinking that twist your interpretation of an event in different ways. This happens commonly in depression. Cognitive behavioral therapy uses a series of exercises to challenge and replace the negative and distorted thoughts that accompany depression.

coping strategies Coping strategies are the steps you can actively take to lessen the effects of stress and decrease your vulnerability to stressors. Coping includes problem solving, self-soothing, relaxation, distraction, humor, mindfulness meditation, and other techniques.

depression Depression is a relapsing and remitting but treatable illness. Relapsing and remitting means that the episodes come and go. Depression affects your thoughts, feelings, behaviors, relationships, activities, interests, and many other aspects of life. It is thought to involve a dysfunction in the network of neurons (brain cells) in the brain. This dysfunction may happen when certain life experiences occur in a susceptible person.

distorted thinking Distortions in your thoughts are errors in thinking that twist your interpretation of an event in different ways. Cognitive behavioral therapy uses a series of exercises to challenge and replace the negative and distorted thoughts that accompany depression.

distress tolerance Distress tolerance is the ability to endure extreme distress for a short period, until the crisis of the moment passes. It is a strategy to get through a brief difficult time when you cannot change the situation. Distress tolerance strategies include using skills to distract yourself, soothe yourself, provide solace, and improve the difficult moment.

metabolic syndrome A physical condition seen in about 40 percent of those who have depression, metabolic syndrome consists of having three of the following five cardiovascular risk factors: central (around the midsection) obesity, high blood pressure, high levels of triglycerides in the blood, low levels of the "good" HDL cholesterol, or high levels of fasting blood sugar. Having metabolic syndrome puts you at increased chance of having a heart attack, stroke, or diabetes.

mood disorders Mood disorders is a term that includes major depression and bipolar disorder, conditions of the brain that involve a disturbance in your mood or state of mind.

psychomotor agitation Psychomotor agitation is a symptom best described as a combination of excessive physical and mental (or cognitive) activity occurring at the same time. It is usually without purpose and is non-productive. This agitation can be a symptom of some mental health conditions, such as in the mania or hypomania of bipolar disorder.

relapse prevention Relapse prevention is an effective daily approach to help you minimize the chance of a relapse, or return of symptoms, and to help you stay well. Relapse prevention means identifying and responding promptly to changes in your warning signs, triggers, or symptoms. This helps you to take steps when an important change in your emotional health may be happening. Early identification and intervention can prevent your episode from worsening.

shared decision making Shared decision making is a process in which you make health care decisions in partnership with your treatment provider. It takes into account your personal goals, preferences, and values.

sleep hygiene Sleep hygiene refers to the personal habits, behaviors, and environmental (home) conditions that can help you get the sleep you need. Attending to these habits can help improve the quality and the quantity of your sleep. It is important to pay attention to sleep hygiene principles during episodes of depression, when your sleep patterns are likely to be disrupted.

triggers Triggers are events or circumstances that may cause you distress and lead to an increase in your symptoms of depression.

warning signs Warning signs are distinct changes from your baseline healthy self that precede an episode of depression or mania.

well-being More than the absence of symptoms, feeling well is having the life skills that bring you satisfaction. It means you feel involved in things greater than yourself. Wellness includes having a sense of realizing your full potential, with improvement over time, having positive relationships, a feeling of independence and being in control of your life, having a sense of competence and mastery, and feeling good about yourself.

References

Introduction

Bodenheimer, T., K. Lorig, H. Holman, et al. Patient self-management of chronic disease in primary care. JAMA 2002;288(19):2469–75.

Ludman, E., W. Katon, T. Bush, et al. Behavioural factors associated with symptom outcomes in a primary care-based depression prevention intervention trial. Psychol Med 2003;33(6):1061–70.

Styron, William. *Darkness Visible: A Memoir of Madness*. New York: Vintage Books, 1990.

Yeung, A., G. Feldman, and M. Fava. *Self-Management of Depression: A Manual for Mental Health and Primary Care Professionals*. New York: Cambridge University Press, 2010.

Chapter 1. Mental Health Basics

Sleep

American Academy of Sleep Medicine. *Healthy Sleep Habits*. Updated February 9, 2017. www.sleepeducation.org/essentials-in-sleep/healthy-sleep-habits.

Goodwin, F. K., and K. R. Jamison. *Manic-Depressive Illness*. 2nd ed. New York: Oxford University Press, 2007.

Tsuno, N., S. Besset, and K. Ritchie. Sleep and depression. J Clin Psychiatry 2005;66(10):1254–69.

US National Institutes of Health and National Heart, Lung, and Blood Institute. *Your Guide to Healthy Sleep*. Bethesda, MD: NHLBI, 2011. www.nhlbi.nih.gov/files/docs/public/sleep/healthy_sleep.pdf.

Winkelman, J. W. Insomnia disorder. N Engl J Med 2015;373(15):1437–44.

Winkelman, J. W., and D. T. Plante, eds. *Foundations of Psychiatric Sleep Medicine*. New York: Cambridge University Press, 2011.

Nutrition

Bodnar, L. M., and K. L. Wisner. Nutrition and depression: Implications for improving mental health among childbearing-aged women. Biol Psych 2005;58(9):679–85.

Fava, M. Weight gain and antidepressants. J Clin Psychiatry 2000;61(suppl 11):37–41.

Hirschfeld, R. M. A. Long-term side effects of SSRI's: Sexual dysfunction and weight gain. J Clin Psychiatry 2003;64(suppl 18):20–24.

Jacka, F. N., J. A. Pasco, A. Mykletun, et al. Association of western and traditional diets with depression and anxiety in women. Am J Psychiatry 2010;167(3):305–11.

Nielsen, S. J., and B. M. Popkin. Patterns and trends in food portion sizes, 1977–1998. JAMA 2003;289(4):450–53.

O'Meara, M. Effect of dietary intake on mood and energy level. Personal communication. April 2016.

Papakostas, G. I. Limitations of contemporary antidepressants: Tolerability. J Clin Psychiatry 2007;68(suppl 10):11–17.

US Department of Agriculture and US Department of Health and Human Services. *Dietary Guidelines for Americans, 2015–2020*. 8th ed. Washington, DC: Government Printing Office, 2015. www.health.gov/dietaryguidelines/2015/guidelines.

Exercise

Babyak, M., J. A. Blumenthal, S. Herman, et al. Exercise treatment for major depression: Maintenance of therapeutic benefit at 10 months. Psychosom Med 2000;62(5):633–38.

Cotman, C. W., N. C. Berchtold, and L. A. Christie. Exercise builds brain health: Key roles of growth factor cascades and inflammation. Trends Neurosci 2007;30(9):464–72.

Dunn, A. L., M. H. Trivedi, J. B. Kampert, et al. Exercise treatment for depression: Efficacy and dose response. Am J Prev Med 2005;28(1):1–8.

Garber, C. E., B. Blissmer, M. R. Deschenes, et al. American College of Sports Medicine Position Stand: Quantity and quality of exercise for developing and maintaining cardiorespiratory, musculoskeletal, and neuromotor fitness in apparently healthy adults: Guidelines for prescribing exercise. Med Sci Sports Exerc 2011;43(7):1334–59.

Gelenberg, A. J., M. P. Freeman, J. C. Markowitz, et al. *Practice Guideline for the Treatment of Patients with Major Depressive Disorder*. 3rd ed. Washington, DC: American Psychiatric Association, October 2010.

Haskell, W. L., I. M. Lee, R. R. Pate, et al. Physical activity and public health: Updated recommendation for adults from the American College of Sports Medicine and the American Heart Association. Circulation 2007;116(9):1081–93.

Mead, G. E., W. Morley, P. Campbell, et al. Exercise for depression. Cochrane Database Syst Rev 2009(3):CD004366.

Ratey, J. J., and E. Hagerman. *Spark: The Revolutionary Science of Exercise and the Brain*. New York: Little, Brown, 2008.

Rethorst, C. D., I. Bernstein, and M. H. Trivedi. Inflammation, obesity and metabolic syndrome in depression: Analysis of the 2009–2010 National Health and Nutrition Examination Survey (NHANES). J Clin Psychiatry 2014;75(12):e1428–32.

Rethorst, C. D., D. M. Landers, C. T. Nagoshi, and J. T. Ross. Efficacy of exercise in reducing depressive symptoms across 5-HTTLPR genotypes. Med Sci Sports Exerc 2010;42(11):2141–47.

Rethorst, C. D., and M. H. Trivedi. Evidence-based recommendations for the prescription of exercise for major depressive disorder. J Psychiatr Pract 2013;19(3):204–12.

Rethorst, C. D., B. M. Wipfli, and D. M. Landers. The antidepressant effects of exercise: A meta-analysis of randomized trials. Sports Med 2009;39(6):491–511.

Sylvia, L. G. *The Wellness Workbook for Bipolar Disorder*. Oakland, CA: New Harbinger, 2015.

Trivedi, M. H., T. L. Greer, T. S. Church, et al. Exercise as an augmentation treatment for nonremitted major depressive disorder: A randomized, parallel dose comparison. J Clin Psychiatry 2011;72(5):677–84.

US Centers for Disease Control and Prevention. *Physical Activity*. Last updated November 1, 2017. www.cdc.gov/physicalactivity.

US Department of Health and Human Services. *Physical Activity Guidelines for Americans*. HHS, 2008. www.health.gov/paguidelines/guidelines.

Yeung, A., G. Feldman, and M. Fava. *Self-Management of Depression: A Manual for Mental Health and Primary Care Professionals*. New York: Cambridge University Press, 2010, chap. 5.

Routine and Structure

Frank, E. Interpersonal and social rhythm therapy: A means of improving depression and preventing relapse in bipolar disorder. J Clin Psychol 2007;63(5):463–73.

Frank, E., S. Hlastala, A. Ritenour, et al. Inducing lifestyle regularity in recovering bipolar disorder patients: Results from the maintenance therapies in bipolar disorder protocol. Biol Psychiatry 1997;41(12):1165–73.

Isolation

Kendler, K. S., J. Myers, and C. A. Prescott. Sex differences in the relationship between social support and risk for major depression: A longitudinal study of opposite-sex twin pairs. Am J Psychiatry 2005;162(2):250–56.

Chapter 2. Mood Disorders

aan het Rot, M., K. A. Collins, J. W. Murrough, et al. Safety and efficacy of repeated-dose intravenous ketamine for treatment-resistant depression. Biol Psychiatry 2010;67(2):139–45.

Al-Harbi, K. S. Treatment resistant depression: Therapeutic trends, challenges, and · future directions. Patient Prefer Adherence 2012;6:369–88.

American Psychiatric Association. *Diagnostic and Statistical Manual of Mental Disorders.* 5th ed. Washington, DC: American Psychiatric Association, 2013.

Andrade, A. C. Intranasal drug delivery in neuropsychiatry: Focus on intranasal ketamine for refractory depression. J Clin Psychiatry 2015;76(5):e628-31.

Beck, A. T., and B. A. Alford. *Depression: Causes and Treatment.* Philadelphia: University of Pennsylvania Press, 2009.

Berlim, M. T., and G. Turecki. Definition, assessment, and staging of treatment-resistant refractory major depression: A review of current concepts and methods. Can J Psychiatry 2007;52(1):46–54.

Conway, C. R., M. S. George, and H. S. Sackeim. Toward an evidence-based, operational definition of treatment-resistant depression: When enough is enough. JAMA Psychiatry 2017;74(1):9–10.

Crowther, A., M. J. Smoski, J. Minkel, et al. Resting-state connectivity predictors of response to psychotherapy in major depressive disorder. Neuropsychopharmacology 2015;40(7):1659–73.

Fava, M., J. E. Alpert, C. N. Carmin, et al. Clinical correlates and symptom patterns of anxious depression among patients with major depressive disorder in STAR*D. Psychol Med 2004;34(7):1299–1308.

Goodwin, F. K., and K. R. Jamison. *Manic-Depressive Illness.* 2nd ed. New York: Oxford University Press, 2007.

Hyde, C. L., M. W. Nagle, C. Tian, et al. Identification of 15 genetic loci associated with risk of major depression in individuals of European descent. Nat Genet 2016;48(9):1031–36. doi:10.1038/ng.3623.

Kendler, K. S., M. Gatz, C. O. Gardner, and N. L. Pedersen. A Swedish national twin study of lifetime major depression. Am J Psychiatry 2006;163(1):109–14.

Lapidus, K. A. B., C. F. Levitch, A. M. Perez, et al. A randomized controlled trial of intranasal ketamine in major depressive disorder. Biol Psychiatry 2014; 76(12):970–76.

MacKinnon, D. F. *Still Down: What to Do When Antidepressants Fail.* Baltimore: Johns Hopkins University Press, 2016.

Marcus, S. A. M., E. A. Young, K. B. Kerber, et al. Gender differences in depression: Findings from the STAR*D study. J Affect Disord 2005;87(2–3):141–50.

Murrough, J. W., D. V. Iosifescu, L. C. Chang, et al. Antidepressant efficacy of ketamine in treatment-resistant major depression: A two-site randomized controlled trial. Am J Psychiatry 2013;170(10):1134–42.

Newport, D. J., L. L. Carpenter, W. M. McDonald, et al. American Psychiatric Association (APA) Council of Research Task Force on Novel Biomarkers and Treatments. Ketamine and other NDMA antagonists. Am J Psychiatry 2015;172(10):950–66.

Nierenberg, A. A., and L. M. DeCecco. Definitions of antidepressant treatment response, remission, nonresponse, partial response, and other relevant outcomes: A focus on treatment-resistant depression. J Clin Psychiatry 2001;62(suppl 16):5–9.

Rush, A. J., M. H. Trivedi, S. R. Wisniewski, et al. Acute and longer-term outcomes in depressed outpatients requiring one or several treatment steps: A STAR*D Report. Am J Psychiatry 2006;163(11):1905–17.

Sanacora, G. M., A. Frye, W. McDonald, et al. American Psychiatric Association (APA) Council of Research Task Force on Novel Biomarkers and Treatments. A consensus statement on the use of ketamine in the treatment of mood disorders. JAMA Psychiatry 2017;74(4):399–405.

Saveanu, R. V., and C. B. Nemeroff. Etiology of depression: Genetic and environmental factors. Psychiatr Clin North Am 2012;35(1):51–71.

Stein, M. B., and J. Sareen. Generalized anxiety disorder. N Engl J Med 2015;373(21): 2059–68.

Sullivan, P. F., M. C. Neale, and K. S. Kendler. Genetic epidemiology of major depression: Review and meta-analysis. Am J Psychiatry 2000;157(10):1552–62.

Trevino, K., S. M. McClintock, N. McDonald Fisher, et al. Defining treatment-resistant depression: A comprehensive review of the literature. Ann Clin Psychiatry 2014; 26(3):222–32.

Trivedi, M. H., A. J. Rush, S. R. Wisniewski, et al. Evaluation of outcomes with citalopram for depression using measurement-based care in STAR*D: Implication for clinical practice. Am J Psychiatry 2006;163(1):28–40.

US National Institutes of Health. Ketamine lifts depression via a byproduct of its metabolism. Press Release, May 4, 2016. www.nimh.nih.gov.

Wan, L.-B., C. F. Levitch, A. M. Perez, et al. Ketamine safety and tolerability in clinical trials for treatment-resistant depression. J Clin Psychiatry 2015;76(3):247–52.

Wilkinson, S. T., and G. Sanacora. Considerations on the off-label use of ketamine as a treatment for mood disorders. JAMA 2017;318(9):793–94. doi:10.100/jama.2017.10697.

Yeung, A., G. Feldman, and M. Fava. *Self-Management of Depression: A Manual for Mental Health and Primary Care Professionals*. New York: Cambridge University Press, 2010.

Depression in Women

Barker, E. D., W. Copeland, B. Maughan, et al. Relative impact of maternal depression and associated risk factors on offspring psychopathology. Br J Psychiatry 2012;200(2):124–29.

Batten, L. A., M. Hernandez, D. J. Pilowsky, et al. Children of treatment-seeking mothers: A comparison with the sequenced treatment alternatives to relieve depression (STAR*D) child study. J Am Acad Child Adolesc Psychiatry 2012;51(11):1185–96.

Dubey, N., J. F. Hoffman, K. Schuebel, et al. The ESC/E(Z) complex, an effector of response to ovarian steroids, manifests an intrinsic difference in cells from women with premenstrual dysphoric disorder. Mol Psychiatry 2017;22(8):1172–84. doi:10:1038.

Pilowsky, D. J., P. J. Wickramme, A. J. Rush, et al. Children of currently depressed mothers: A STAR*D ancillary study. J Clin Psychiatry 2006;67(1):126–36.

Schmidt, P. J., R. Ben Dor, P. E. Martinez, et al. Effects of estradiol withdrawal on mood in women with past perimenopausal depression: A randomized clinical trial. JAMA Psychiatry 2015;72(7):714–26.

Sichel, D., and J. W. Driscoll. *Women's Mood's: What Every Woman Must Know about Hormones, the Brain, and Emotional Health.* New York: Quill, 1999.

Stewart, D. E., and S. Vigod. Postpartum depression. N Engl J Med 2016;375(22):2177–85.

US National Institutes of Health. Sex hormone-sensitive gene complex linked to premenstrual mood disorder. Press Release, January 3, 2017. www.nimh.nih.gov.

Depression in Men

Martin, L. A., H. W. Neighbors, and D. M. Griffith. The experience of symptoms of depression in men vs women: Analysis of the National Comorbidity Survey replication. JAMA Psychiatry 2013;70(10):1100–106.

Fatigue and Depression

Arnold, L. M. Understanding fatigue in major depressive disorder and other medical disorders. Psychosomatics 2008;49(3):185–90.

Baldwin, D. S., and G. I. Papakostas. Symptoms of fatigue and sleepiness in major depressive disorder. J Clin Psych 2006;67(suppl 6):9–15.

Nierenberg, A. A., M. M. Husain, M. H. Trivedi, et al. Residual symptoms after remission of major depressive disorder with citalopram and risk of relapse: A STAR*D report. Psychol Med 2010;40(1):41–50.

Nierenberg, A. A., B. R. Keefe, V. C. Leslie, et al. Residual symptoms in depressed patients who respond acutely to fluoxetine. J Clin Psych 1999;60(4):221–25.

Tylee, A., M. Gastpar, J.-P. Lepine, et al., on behalf of the DEPRES Steering Committee. DEPRES II (Depression Research in European Society II): A patient survey of the symptoms, disability and current management of depression in the community. Int Clin Psychopharmacol 1999;14(3):139–51.

Chapter 3. Common Obstacles in Depression

Substance Abuse and Mental Health Services Administration (SAMHSA). Recovery and Recovery Support. Last updated September 20, 2017. www.samhsa.gov/recovery.

Chapter 5. Managing Your Mood Disorder

Beck, A. T., and B. A. Alford. *Depression: Causes and Treatment.* Philadelphia: University of Pennsylvania Press, 2009.

Fava, G. A., C. Rafanelli, S. Grandi, et al. Prevention of recurrent depression with cognitive behavioral therapy: Preliminary findings. Arch Gen Psychiatry 1998;55(9):816–20.

Goodwin, F. K., and K. R. Jamison. *Manic-Depressive Illness.* 2nd ed. New York: Oxford University Press, 2007.

Harley, R., S. Sprich, J. M. Safran, and M. Fava. Adaptation of dialectical behavioral therapy skills training group for treatment-resistant depression. J Nerv Ment Dis 2008;196(2):136–43.

Joint Commission. The Joint Commission launches educational campaign on adult depression. News Release, May 21, 2013.

Lin, E. H. B., M. Von Korff, E. J. Ludman, et al. Enhancing adherence to prevent depression relapse in primary care. Gen Hosp Psychiatry 2003;25(3):303–10.

Linehan, M. M. *Cognitive-Behavioral Treatment of Borderline Personality Disorder*. New York: Guilford Press, 1993.

Ludman, E., W. Katon, T. Bush, et al. Behavioural factors associated with symptom outcomes in a primary care-based depression prevention intervention trial. Psychol Med 2003;33(6):1061–70.

Nierenberg, A. A., T. J. Petersen, and J. A. Alpert. Prevention of relapse and recurrence in depression: The role of long-term pharmacotherapy and psychotherapy. J Clin Psychiatry 2003;64(suppl 15):13–17.

Paykel, E. S., J. Scott, J. D. Teasdale, et al. Prevention of relapse in residual depression by cognitive therapy: A controlled trial. Arch Gen Psychiatry 1999;56(9):829–35.

Petersen, T. J. Enhancing the efficacy of antidepressants with psychotherapy. J Psychopharmacol 2006;20(suppl 3):19–28.

Richards, C. S., and M. G. Perri, ed. *Relapse Prevention for Depression*. Washington, DC: American Psychological Association, 2010.

Simon, G. E., E. H. B. Lin, W. Katon, et al. Outcomes of "inadequate" antidepressant treatment. J Gen Intern Med 1995;10(12):663–70.

Teasdale, J. D., Z. V. Segal, J. M. G. Williams, et al. Prevention of relapse/recurrence in major depression by mindfulness-based cognitive therapy. J Consult Clin Psychol 2000;68(4):615–23.

Trivedi, M. H., E. H. B. Lin, and W. J. Katon. Consensus recommendations for improving adherence, self-management, and outcomes in patients with depression. CNS Spectr 2007;12(8 suppl 13):1–27.

Yeung, A., G. Feldman, and M. Fava. *Self-Management of Depression: A Manual for Mental Health and Primary Care Professionals*. New York: Cambridge University Press, 2010.

Chapter 6. What Is the Goal?

Ryff, C. D. Psychological well-being revisited: Advances in science and practice. Psychother Psychosom 2014;83(1):10–28.

Sylvia, L. G. *The Wellness Workbook for Bipolar Disorder*. Oakland, CA: New Harbinger, 2015.

Chapter 7. Relapse Prevention

American Psychiatric Association. *Diagnostic and Statistical Manual of Mental Disorders*. 5th ed. Washington, DC: American Psychiatric Association, 2013.

Beck, A. T., and B. A. Alford. *Depression: Causes and Treatment*. Philadelphia: University of Pennsylvania Press, 2009.

Fava, G. A., C. Rafanelli, S. Grandi, et al. Prevention of recurrent depression with cognitive behavioral therapy. Arch Gen Psychiatry 1998;55(9):816–20.

Frank, E. Interpersonal and social rhythm therapy: A means of improving depression and preventing relapse in bipolar disorder. J Clin Psychol 2007;63(5):463–73.

Frank, E., S. Hlastala, A. Ritenour, et al. Inducing lifestyle regularity in recovering bipolar disorder patients: Results from the maintenance therapies in bipolar disorder protocol. Biol Psychiatry 1997;41(12):1165–73.

Ludman, E., W. Katon, T. Bush, et al. Behavioural factors associated with symptom outcomes in a primary care-based depression prevention intervention trial. Psychol Med 2003;33(6):1061–70.

Paykel, E. S., J. Scott, J. D. Teasdale, et al. Prevention of relapse in residual depression by cognitive therapy: A controlled trial. Arch Gen Psychiatry 1999;56(9):829–35.

Petersen, T. J. Enhancing the efficacy of antidepressants with psychotherapy. J Psychopharmacol 2006;20(suppl 3):19–28.

Richards, C. S., and M. G. Perri, eds. *Relapse Prevention for Depression*. Washington, DC: American Psychological Association, 2010.

Teasdale, J. D., Z. V. Segal, J. M. G. Williams, et al. Prevention of relapse/recurrence in major depression by mindfulness-based cognitive therapy. J Consult Clin Psychol 2000;68(4):615–23.

Chapter 8. Cognitive Behavioral Therapy

Beck, A. T., and B. A. Alford. *Depression: Causes and Treatment*. Philadelphia: University of Pennsylvania Press, 2009.

Beck, A. T., A. J. Rush, B. F. Shaw, and G. Emery. *Cognitive Therapy of Depression*. New York: Guilford Press, 1979.

Burns, David. *Feeling Good: The New Mood Therapy*. New York: Avon Books, 1980.

Goodwin, F. K., and K. R. Jamison. *Manic-Depressive Illness*. 2nd ed. New York: Oxford University Press, 2007.

Sudak, D. M. Cognitive behavioral therapy for depression. Psychiatr Clin North Am 2012;35(1):99–110.

Chapter 9. Strategies to Get You through the Tough Times

Benson, Herbert. *The Relaxation Response*. Rev. ed. New York: Harper, 2000.

Styron, William. *Darkness Visible: A Memoir of Madness*. New York: Vintage Books, 1990.

Mindfulness

Kabat-Zinn, Jon. *Wherever You Go, There You Are*. New York: Hyperion, 1994.

Linehan, M. M. *Skills Training Manual for Treating Borderline Personality Disorder*. New York: Guilford Press, 1993.

Mindfulness: The New Science of Health and Happiness. New York: Time Special Edition, 2017.

Segal, Z. V., J. M. G. Williams, and J. D. Teasdale. *Mindfulness-Based Cognitive Therapy for Depression*. New York: Guilford Press, 2002.

Distress Tolerance

Linehan, M. M. *Cognitive-Behavioral Treatment of Borderline Personality Disorder*. New York: Guilford Press, 1993.

Linehan, M. M. *Skills Training Manual for Treating Borderline Personality Disorder*. New York: Guilford Press, 1993.

Communication Skills

Booher, Dianna. *Communicate with Confidence: How to Say It Right the First Time*. New York: McGraw-Hill, 1994.

Davidson, Jeff. *The Complete Idiot's Guide to Assertiveness*. New York: Alpha Books, 1997.

Fine, Debra. *The Fine Art of Small Talk*. New York: Hyperion, 2005.

Yeung, A., G. Feldman, and M. Fava. *Self-Management of Depression: A Manual for Mental Health and Primary Care Professionals*. New York: Cambridge University Press, 2010, app. C.

Chapter 10. Dealing with Family and Friends

Sylvia, L. G. *The Wellness Workbook for Bipolar Disorder*. Oakland, CA: New Harbinger, 2015.

Chapter 12. Collective Wisdom

American Psychological Association. *What You Need to Know before Choosing Online Therapy*. Washington, DC: American Psychological Association, 2017.

Areán, Patricia. A BRIGHT technological future for mental health trials: The BRIGHTEN study. Science Update, February 19, 2016. www.nimh.nih.gov/news/science-news /2016/a-bright-technological-future-for-mental-health-trials.shtml.

Christensen, H. K., M. Griffiths, and A. Korten. Web-based cognitive behavior therapy: Analysis of site usage and changes in depression and anxiety scores. J Med Internet Res 2002;4(1):e3.

Firth, J., J. Torous, J. Nicholas, et al. The efficacy of smartphone-based mental health interventions for depressive symptoms: A meta-analysis of randomized controlled trials. World Psychiatry 2017;16(3):287–98.

Franklin, J. C., K. R. Fox, C. R. Franklin, et al. A brief mobile app reduces nonsuicidal and suicidal self-injury: Evidence from three randomized controlled trials. J Consult Clin Psychol 2016 ;84(6):544–57.

Harrison, V., J. Proudfoot, P. P. Wee, et al. Mobile mental health: Review of the emerging field and proof of concept study. J Ment Health 2011;20(6):509–24.

Index